Mastering DALK

A Video Textbook on Deep Anterior Lamellar Keratoplasty

Mastering DALK

A Video Textbook on Deep Anterior Lamellar Keratoplasty

Edited by

Soosan Jacob, MS, FRCS, DNB, MNAMS
Director and Chief
Dr. Agarwal's Refractive and Cornea Foundation
Dr. Agarwal's Group of Eye Hospitals
Chennai, India

SLACK
INCORPORATED

SLACK
INCORPORATED

SLACK Incorporated
6900 Grove Road
Thorofare, NJ 08086 USA
856-848-1000 Fax: 856-848-6091
www.Healio.com/books

Senior Vice President: Stephanie Arasim Portnoy
Vice President, Editorial: Jennifer Kilpatrick
Vice President, Marketing: Michelle Gatt
Acquisitions Editor: Tony Schiavo
Managing Editor: Allegra Tiver
Creative Director: Thomas Cavallaro
Cover Artist: Lori Shields
Project Editor: Emily Densten

The procedures and practices described in this publication should be implemented in a manner consistent with the professional standards set for the circumstances that apply in each specific situation. Every effort has been made to confirm the accuracy of the information presented and to correctly relate generally accepted practices. The authors, editors, and publisher cannot accept responsibility for errors or exclusions or for the outcome of the material presented herein. There is no expressed or implied warranty of this book or information imparted by it. Care has been taken to ensure that drug selection and dosages are in accordance with currently accepted/recommended practice. Off-label uses of drugs may be discussed. Due to continuing research, changes in government policy and regulations, and various effects of drug reactions and interactions, it is recommended that the reader carefully review all materials and literature provided for each drug, especially those that are new or not frequently used. Some drugs or devices in this publication have clearance for use in a restricted research setting by the Food and Drug and Administration or FDA. Each professional should determine the FDA status of any drug or device prior to use in their practice.

Any review or mention of specific companies or products is not intended as an endorsement by the author or publisher.

SLACK Incorporated uses a review process to evaluate submitted material. Prior to publication, educators or clinicians provide important feedback on the content that we publish. We welcome feedback on this work.

Library of Congress Cataloging-in-Publication Data
Names: Jacob, Soosan, editor.
Title: Mastering DALK : a video textbook on deep anterior lamellar keratoplasty / editor, Soosan Jacob.
Description: Thorofare, NJ : SLACK Incorporated, [2019] | Includes bibliographical references and index.
Identifiers: LCCN 2018047696 (print) | LCCN 2018048458 (ebook) | ISBN 9781630914578 (epub) | ISBN 9781630914585 (web) | ISBN 9781630914561 (alk. paper)
Subjects: | MESH: Corneal Transplantation--methods
Classification: LCC RE336 (ebook) | LCC RE336 (print) | NLM WW 220 | DDC 617.7/190592--dc23
LC record available at https://lccn.loc.gov/2018047696

Printed in the United States of America.

Last digit is print number: 10 9 8 7 6 5 4 3 2 1

Dedication

"The love of a family is life's greatest blessing."—Eva Burrows

This book is dedicated to my family
My husband, Dr. Abraham Oomman
My children, Ashwin and Riya Abraham
My parents, Lt. Col. Jacob Mathai and Mrs. Mary Jacob
My parents-in-law, Mr. MC Oomman and Mrs. Annamma Oomman
My brothers and sister, Col. Alex Jacob, Dr. Asha Varghese, and
Mr. Bejoy George Oomman
All of whom are God's best gifts to me ever!!

Contents

Acknowledgments

I would like to thank many people for making this book possible. My co-authors who contributed valuable time and effort toward excellent text, pictures, and high-quality narrated videos and my friends and colleagues for their constant support. I would also like to thank Tony Schiavo from SLACK Incorporated for encouraging me to take on this task, for keeping me at it to complete it and for helping keep the book to such high standards; Julia Dolinger, Kayla Whittle, Allegra Tiver, Emily Densten and the rest of the team from SLACK Incorporated for being immensely helpful at every step; Areeckal Incy Saijimol for helping me organize things better and make my life easier; and of course, all my patients from whom I have learned so much and all the teachers in my life who have taught me so much. I would like to especially thank Drs. Amar and Athiya Agarwal who have been my mentors and always pushed me forwards.

Last but not the least, I would like to thank ***my family****—my parents, Lt. Col. Jacob Mathai and Mrs. Mary Jacob, for guiding me and molding me into what I am; my brother Col. Alex Jacob and my sister Dr. Asha Varghese for always being there for me; and most of all, my husband, Dr. Abraham Oomman—my best friend, confidante, and sounding board for his unflinching support, constant love and encouragement to keep raising the bar further and further; and lastly my children, Ashwin and Riya Abraham, who tolerate me throughout and keep me smiling through all the long hours spent.*

About the Editor

Soosan Jacob, MS, FRCS, DNB, MNAMS is Director and Chief, Dr. Agarwal's Refractive and Cornea Foundation (DARCF) and Senior Consultant, Cataract and Glaucoma Services, Dr. Agarwal's Group of Eye Hospitals, Chennai, India. She is a noted speaker, widely respected for her innovative techniques and management of complex surgical scenarios. She conducts courses and delivers lectures in numerous national and international conferences; has been the recipient of Intraocular Implant and Refractive Society of India Special Gold Medal, *Journal of Refractive Surgery* (JRS) Waring Medal for Editorial Excellence, International Society of Refractive Surgery (ISRS) Kritzinger Memorial award, Connecticut Society of Eye Physicians Innovator's award, European Society of Cataract and Refractive Surgeons (ESCRS) John Henahan Award for Young Ophthalmologist, American Academy of Ophthalmology (AAO) International Ophthalmologist Education award, AAO International Scholar award, AAO Achievement award, American Society of Cataract and Refractive Surgery (ASCRS) Top-Gun Instructor award, Uttarakhand State Ophthalmological Society gold medal, AM Gokhale award and oration, Bruce Jackson oration, Harold Stein Innovator lecture, of ASCRS Golden Apple award two times. In addition, she has won more than 50 prestigious international awards for her surgical videos on her innovations and challenging cases at prestigious international conferences in the United States and Europe. She has authored more than 100 peer-reviewed publications, more than 200 chapters in 34 textbooks, and is editor for 17 ophthalmology textbooks and reviewer for many prestigious journals. She is Chair of the Multimedia Editorial Board American Academy of Ophthalmology-International Society of Refractive Surgery, associate editor—*Journal of Refractive Surgery*, Section Editor (Refractive Surgery)—*EyeNet* (American Academy of Ophthalmology, is on the editorial board of *International Journal of Ophthalmology*, *EyeNet* (AAO), *EuroTimes*, *International Journal of Keratoconus and Ectatic Corneal Diseases*, *Ocular Surgery News-Asia Pacific*, *Glaucoma Today*, *Cataract & Refractive Surgery Today Europe*, *Journal of Ophthalmic Science and Research*, and *Ophthalmology & Therapy*, and is a member ISRS Executive Committee.

She has special interest in cutting-edge cataract, cornea, glaucoma, complex anterior segment reconstruction, and refractive surgery. Her innovations, many of which have won international awards, include: anterior segment transplantation, where cornea, sclera, artificial iris, pupil, and intraocular lens are transplanted en bloc for anterior staphyloma; suprabrow single-stab incision ptosis surgery to enhance postoperative cosmesis; turnaround techniques for false channel dissection during Intacs (Addition Technology, Inc) implantation; glued endocapsular ring, glued capsular hook, and the paper clip capsule stabilizer for subluxated cataracts; stab incision glaucoma surgery (SIGS) as a guarded filtration surgery technique; contact lens–assisted corneal cross-linking (CACXL) for safely cross-linking thin keratoconic corneas; endo-illuminator–assisted Descemet's membrane endothelial keratoplasty, air pump–assisted pre-Descemet's endothelial keratoplasty, and host Descemetic scaffolding for easier and better surgical results; presbyopic allogenic refractive lenticule (PEARL) inlay for treating presbyopia, corneal allogeneic intrastromal ring segment (CAIRS) for keratoconus and other corneal ectasias; the Jacob modified technique for pre-Descemetic deep anterior lamellar keratoplasty (DALK) as a primary treatment for acute hydrops; sutureless small incision lenticule extraction (SMILE) lenticule-assisted resurfacing with interface tattooing for limbal dermoid and peripheral corneal scars; and white ring sign and the sequential segmental terminal lenticular side cut dissection for safe and effective lenticule extraction in SMILE surgery. She has proposed a new classification of Descemet's membrane detachments into rhegmatogenous, tractional, bullous, and complex detachments with a suitable treatment algorithm and a new technique of relaxing descemetotomy for tractional Descemet's detachment.

Her surgeries and surgical techniques have often been Editor's Choice in prestigious international ophthalmic websites, such as AAO/ONE network, ISRS, and Eyetube. She has two popular bimonthly columns, "Complications in Cataract and Refractive Surgery" and "Everything You Want to Know About" in the prestigious *EuroTimes* magazine published by ESCRS. She is also the first surgeon internationally to be featured in a dedicated webpage by the *EuroTimes*. She has her own surgical educational YouTube channel, Dr. Soosan Jacob, with more than 8000 subscribers. Her video blog "Journey into the Eye—A Surgeon's Video Blog" in the prestigious *Ocular Surgery News*, USA and her Facebook pages also feature her surgical videos. Dr. Jacob is senior faculty for training postgraduate, fellowship, and overseas doctors.

Her life and work have been featured on the *Ocular Surgery News* cover page, "5Q" interview (prestigious Cataract and Refractive Surgery Today [CRST]), "Sound Off" column (CRST), and "One Day in the Life of..." (CRST). She is also the first researcher internationally to be interviewed in the prestigious CRST "Researcher's Column."

Contributing Authors

Sriram Annavajjhala, MBBS, DOMS (DNB) (Chapter 1)
Rajan Eye Care Hospital Pvt Ltd
Chennai, India

Harkaran S. Bains, BHSc Oph (Chapter 5)
Sight By Design
Edmonton, Alberta, Canada

Rénuka S. Birbal, MD (Chapter 7)
Netherlands Institute for Innovative Ocular Surgery
Melles Cornea Clinic
Amnitrans EyeBank
Rotterdam, Netherlands

Alan N. Carlson, MD (Chapter 3)
Professor
Department of Ophthalmology
Duke University School of Medicine
Durham, North Carolina

Melissa B. Daluvoy, MD (Chapter 3)
Assistant Professor of Ophthalmology
Duke University School of Medicine
Cornea, Refractive and External Disease Fellowship Director
Duke University Eye Center
Durham, North Carolina

Vittoria De Rosa, MD (Chapter 2)
Department of Medico-Surgical Sciences and Biotechnology
Sapienza University of Rome
Latina, Italy

Alaa M. Eldanasoury, MD (Chapter 5)
Magrabi Eye Hospital
Jeddah, Saudia Arabia

Ronald N. Gaster, MD, FACS (Chapter 11)
Clinical Professor of Ophthalmology.
Gavin Herbert Eye Institute
University of California, Irvine
Irvine, California
Cornea Eye Institute
Beverly Hills, California

Noopur Gupta, MBBS, MS, DNB, PhD (Chapter 4)
Cornea, Cataract and Refractive Surgery Services
Dr. Rajendra Prasad Centre for Ophthalmic Sciences
All India Institute of Medical Science
New Delhi, India

Kristin E. Hirabayashi, MD (Chapter 8)
Byers Eye Institute
Stanford University
Palo Alto, California

Bina John, MBBS, DNB, FRCS (Chapter 1)
Rajan Eye Care Hospital
Chennai, India

Terry Kim, MD (Chapter 3)
Professor of Ophthalmology
Duke University School of Medicine
Chief, Cornea and External and Disease Division
Director, Refractive Surgery Service
Duke University Eye Center
Durham, North Carolina

Lim Li, MBBS, FRCS(Ed), MMed(Ophth), FAMS(S'pore) (Video Appendix)
Senior Consultant
Corneal and External Eye Disease
Singapore National Eye Centre
Singapore

Charles C. Lin, MD (Chapter 8)
Clinical Assistant Professor
Cornea Fellowship Director
Byers Eye Institute
Stanford University
Palo Alto, California

Prafulla Maharana, MD (Chapter 10)
Dr. Rajendra Prasad Centre for Ophthalmic Sciences
All India Institute of Medical Sciences
New Delhi, India

Gerrit R. J. Melles, MD, PhD (Chapter 7)
Netherlands Institute for Innovative Ocular Surgery
Melles Cornea Clinic
Amnitrans EyeBank
Rotterdam, Netherlands

Sujatha Mohan, MBBS, DO, MCh, FRCS, FACS (Chapter 1)
Phaco Refractive Cornea Surgeon
Rajan Eye Care Hospital/Rajan Eye Bank
Chennai, India

Smita Narasimhan, MBBS (Chapter 12)
Dr. Agarwal's Refractive and Cornea Foundation
Chennai, India

Ashiyana Nariani, MD, MPH (Chapter 3)
Clinical Associate
Cornea and Refractive Surgery
Duke University Eye Center
Durham, North Carolina

Jack Parker, MD, PhD (Chapter 7)
Netherlands Institute for Innovative Ocular Surgery
Rotterdam, Netherlands
Parker Cornea
Birmingham, Alabama

Mukesh Patil, MBBS, MD, FICO, FAICO (Chapter 4)
Ex-Senior Resident
Dr. Rajendra Prasad Centre for Ophthalmic Sciences
All India Institute of Medical Sciences
New Delhi, India

Claudia Perez-Straziota, MD (Chapter 11)
Assistant Clinical Professor
University of Southern California
Cornea Eye Institute
Beverly Hills, California

Pranita Sahay, MD (Chapter 10)
Dr. Rajendra Prasad Centre for Ophthalmic Sciences
All India Institute of Medical Sciences
New Delhi, India

Areeckal Incy Saijimol, BSc (Chapter 9)
Dr. Agarwal's Refractive and Cornea Foundation
Dr. Agarwal's Eye Hospital and Eye Research Centre
Chennai, India

Namrata Sharma, MD (Chapter 10)
Dr. Rajendra Prasad Centre for Ophthalmic Sciences
All India Institute of Medical Sciences
New Delhi, India

Deepali Singhal, MD, DNB, FICO, FICO (Chapter 10)
Senior Resident
Cornea, Cataract and Refractive Surgery Services
Dr. Rajendra Prasad Centre for Ophthalmic Sciences
All India Institute of Medical Science
New Delhi, India

T. Suchi Smitha, MS, DNB, FCRS (Chapter 6)
Deenanath Mangeshkar Hospital
Pune, India

Leopoldo Spadea, MD (Chapter 2)
Department of Sensory Organs
Head, Eye Clinic
Policlinico Umberto 1
Sapienza University of Rome
Rome, Italy

Rishi Swarup, FRCS (Chapter 6)
Swarup Eye Centre
Hyderabad, India

Radhika Tandon, MBBS, MD, DNB, MNAMS, FRCS(Ed), FRCOphth, MNASI (Chapter 4)
Professor of Ophthalmology
Dr. Rajendra Prasad Centre for Ophthalmic Sciences
All India Institute of Medical Sciences
New Delhi, India

Sherif Said Tolees, FRCS (Chapter 5)
Magrabi Eye Hospital
Jeddah, Saudi Arabia

C. Maya Tong, BSc, MD (Chapter 7)
Netherlands Institute for Innovative Ocular Surgery
Rotterdam, Netherlands
University of Alberta
Edmonton, Alberta, Canada

Korine van Dijk, BOptom, PhD (Chapter 7)
Netherlands Institute for Innovative Ocular Surgery
Melles Cornea Clinic
Rotterdam, Netherlands

Murugesan Vanathi, MBBS, MD (Chapter 4)
Professor of Ophthalmology
Cornea, Cataract and Refractive Services
Dr. Rajendra Prasad Centre for Ophthalmic Sciences
All India Institute of Medical Sciences
New Delhi, India

Preface

Keratoconus is a condition that is not only widely prevalent but is also increasingly being identified with the advent of newer diagnostic technologies. With the inclusion of corneal cross-linking (CXL) and its rapid uptake by practitioners, the good news is that many patients are prevented from going into the more advanced stages of keratoconus that would otherwise require corneal transplantation. However, there are still a large number of patients worldwide who have disease advanced enough to require deep anterior lamellar keratoplasty (DALK). In addition, there are many other indications where an anterior lamellar keratoplasty, whether superficial or deep, may be indicated. Despite the well-known and documented advantages of anterior lamellar keratoplasty when compared to a penetrating keratoplasty, there is a definite delay in widespread adoption of surgical procedures, such as superficial anterior lamellar keratoplasty and DALK, by corneal surgeons. This is because of a perceived steeper learning curve and demand for greater surgical skill. This book is an attempt to bridge this gap and make lamellar keratoplasty easy to adopt by familiarizing the surgeon with indications, surgical steps, postoperative care, and avoidance, as well as management of any complications, thus giving him or her the required capabilities to perform this surgery without dread or fear. It covers all major topics in lamellar keratoplasty and is aimed to be a thorough and comprehensive guide for both the beginner and the established corneal surgeon. There are numerous accompanying high-quality photos and an impressive compendium of narrated surgical videos that aim at making this book unique and very valuable. The contributors, all well-versed in superficial and deep anterior lamellar keratoplasty techniques, share their valuable knowledge in performing surgeries ranging from the straightforward to the very challenging cases and do an excellent job of presenting advantages and disadvantages of each technique in a balanced fashion and without any bias. The book also refers to the techniques of small incision lenticule extraction (SMILE) lenticule-assisted corneal resurfacing with interface tattooing for limbal dermoids and peripheral corneal scars, as well as corneal allogeneic intrastromal ring segments (CAIRS) in certain advanced cases of keratoconus. It also explains the newly introduced Jacob modified technique of pre-Descemetic DALK as immediate primary treatment of acute hydrops in order to avoid scarring.

An attempt has been made to present information in an organized manner that is easy to follow and reference. I hope this book will help in demystifying and decoding lamellar keratoplasty, especially DALK, in a step-by-step and lucid manner, thereby making it easier for ophthalmic surgeons, be they beginners or established, who wish to expand their armamentarium. Not only cornea specialists, but also general ophthalmologists as well as residents and fellows, would find this interesting as they can learn about indications for surgery, choice of surgery, and postoperative management in order to make the appropriate recommendations, referrals, and treatment plans for patients.

Finally, as Herbert Spencer said, "The great aim of education is not knowledge but action."

I hope this book will encourage each reader to adopt anterior lamellar keratoplasty techniques and management protocols into his or her practice. I hope you, the reader, will enjoy this book and find it invaluable.

Soosan Jacob, MS, FRCS, DNB, MNAMS
Director and Chief
Dr. Agarwal's Refractive and Cornea Foundation
Dr. Agarwal's Group of Eye Hospitals
Chennai, India

FOREWORD

The field of surgical cornea has recently undergone a renaissance, moving from traditional penetrating keratoplasty (PK) to selective lamellar keratoplasty as well as other reconstructive procedures. Indeed now, almost any patient who would normally have been offered a PK 25 years ago could be offered something else today, including endothelial keratoplasty (EK) for endothelial dysfunction, deep anterior lamellar keratoplasty (DALK) for stromal opacities, keratoprosthesis for multiple graft failures, and even femtosecond laser–assisted PK if a re-graft is warranted and other procedures are not indicated.

Although EK has become the standard of care for treating isolated endothelial dysfunction, DALK has not been as readily adopted. This is due in part to the numerous advancements and innovations in techniques that have helped corneal surgeons produce reliable and consistent surgical results for their EK patients. On the other hand, techniques for performing DALK, while good, have not necessarily been widespread enough to allow for surgeons to achieve the consistent outcomes that they demand. *Mastering DALK: A Video Textbook on Deep Anterior Lamellar Keratoplasty*, edited by Dr. Soosan Jacob, is written with the intention to change this.

Dr. Jacob is an international authority in corneal surgery. As a widely-honored corneal surgeon, she has also been the innovator and developer of many surgical techniques that have advanced and revolutionized our field, including many in the area of keratoconus and DALK. For this textbook, Dr. Jacob has assembled a team of esteemed corneal surgeons to help make DALK a highly successful procedure for every corneal surgeon. She has carefully organized the textbook to include coverage of the basics of DALK, beginning with correct patient selection and when to do DALK as opposed to PK. Techniques for performing various types of DALK are then described in detail, using high-quality instructive videos to guide the reader. More advanced situations that may be amenable to DALK are then discussed, and the textbook concludes with important tips on how to prevent and manage complications. She has also introduced topics such as corneal allogeneic intrastromal ring segments (CAIRS) and contact lens–assisted corneal cross-linking (CACXL) in order to avoid a DALK in some situations. The unique aspect of this textbook is the videos: one cannot just read about corneal surgical techniques, or even just look at intraoperative photographs. The videos in this textbook bring DALK to life, and the instructors have captured the essence of the techniques in a manner to allow the viewer to easily understand exactly what needs to be done.

With this video textbook, Dr. Jacob has made a big step forward in helping to train cornea surgeons around the world in performing DALK. It is my hope, and indeed my anticipation, that this textbook will help the world's corneal surgeons to offer and to perform DALK for their patients and be able to provide them with consistently outstanding surgical outcomes. In turn, this will allow the patients to enjoy the benefits of undergoing DALK.

Bennie H. Jeng, MD
Department of Ophthalmology and Visual Sciences
University of Maryland School of Medicine
Baltimore, Maryland

1

History of Anterior Lamellar Keratoplasty

Sujatha Mohan, MBBS, DO, MCh, FRCS, FACS;
Bina John, MBBS, DNB, FRCS; and
Sriram Annavajjhala, MBBS, DOMS (DNB)

Early History of Corneal Transplantation

The history of corneal transplantation can be traced as far back as the 2nd century AD when the Greek physician Galen (130–200 AD) proposed abrasiocor'naea (precursor of superficial keratectomy) as a means of restoring corneal transparency.[1] From then to the 17th century can be called the *Dark Ages of corneal transplantation* when there were no reports regarding any significant progress as far as corneal experimentation and research are concerned. In the 18th century, the French surgeon Guillame Pellier de Quengsy published a monograph where he suggested that an opaque cornea could be replaced by a transparent material to restore vision.[2]

The blinding Egyptian ophthalmia (trachoma) of the early 19th century led to experiments with corneal transplantation from the initial work of Samuel Bigger who did the first successful allograft in a gazelle in the year 1837[3] and Richard Kissam, who replaced a young Irishman's opaque cornea with a xenograft from a pig in the year 1838.[4] The rest of the 19th century saw divided opinions among ophthalmologists between those who favored allografts to xenografts and also between lamellar and full-thickness keratoplasties.

The first successful human allograft transplantation was performed in 1905 by Edward Zirm, who transplanted a donor cornea from the enucleated eye of an 11-year-old with penetrating injury to a patient with bilateral alkali burns.[5] The Russian ophthalmologist Vladimir Filatov (1875–1956) was the first to suggest the use of cadaver eyes for corneal transplants.[6] Penetrating keratoplasty (PK) had been

Jacob S, ed. *Mastering DALK: A Video Textbook on Deep Anterior Lamellar Keratoplasty* (pp 1-8).

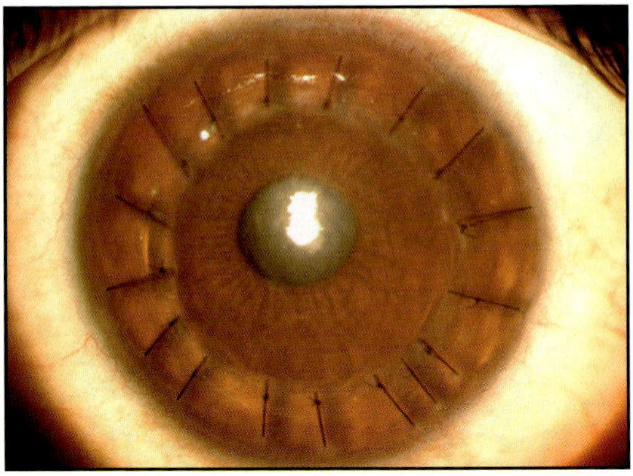

Figure 1-1. Penetrating keratoplasty. (Reprinted with permission from Dr. Soosan Jacob, Dr. Agarwal's Eye Hospital, Chennai, India.)

the gold standard for corneal transplantation from then until the end of the 20th century (Figure 1-1). However, PK with its attendant problems of intraoperative complications secondary to the open-sky technique and postoperative problems, including glaucoma, uveitis, cataract, cystoid macular edema, surface irregularity, and astigmatism, led to research into a suitable alternative to PK, leading to the beginnings of lamellar keratoplasty (LK), which is now slowly replacing PK as the surgery of choice in patients with corneal opacities (Figure 1-2).

Lamellar Keratoplasty

Selective transplantation of diseased layers of the cornea is performed while retaining healthy tissue. It can be either anterior or posterior LK depending on whether the anterior or posterior corneal layers are transplanted based on the site of corneal pathology.

Anterior Lamellar Keratoplasty

Anterior lamellar keratoplasty (ALK) involves removal of diseased corneal tissue leaving behind healthy stroma, Descemet's membrane (DM), or endothelium. ALK is indicated for disorders with a healthy endothelium, such as keratoconus, superficial scars, and anterior corneal dystrophies. ALK can be superficial anterior lamellar keratoplasty (SALK) or deep anterior lamellar keratoplasty (DALK).

Superficial Anterior Lamellar Keratoplasty

SALK is performed when the anterior 30% to 50% of the cornea is affected and replaced with a similar amount of donor tissue. Stroma-to-stroma interface may, however, lead to degradation of visual acuity over time.[7]

Deep Anterior Lamellar Keratoplasty

In DALK where the recipient cornea is dissected up to the DM, the stroma-DM interface is reported to have better visual results[8,9] (Figure 1-3).

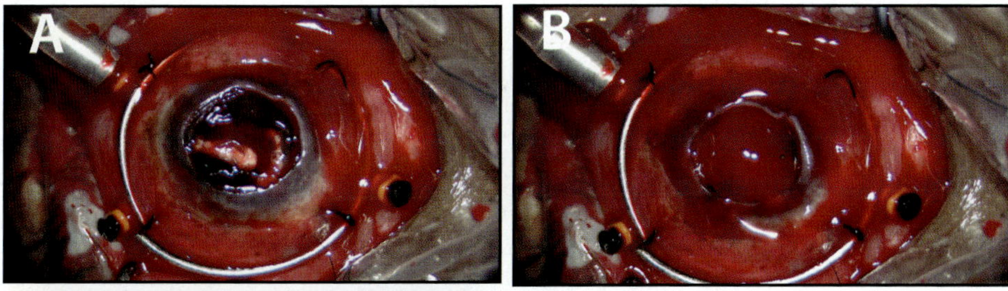

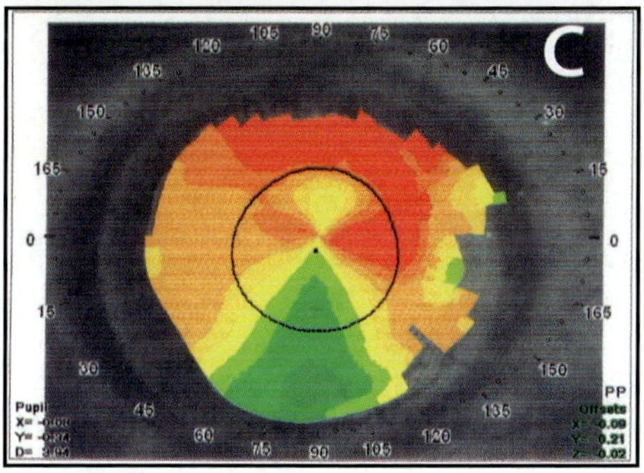

Figure 1-2. (A, B) Expulsive hemorrhage in open-sky procedure. (C) Post-PK with irregular astigmatism on corneal topography.

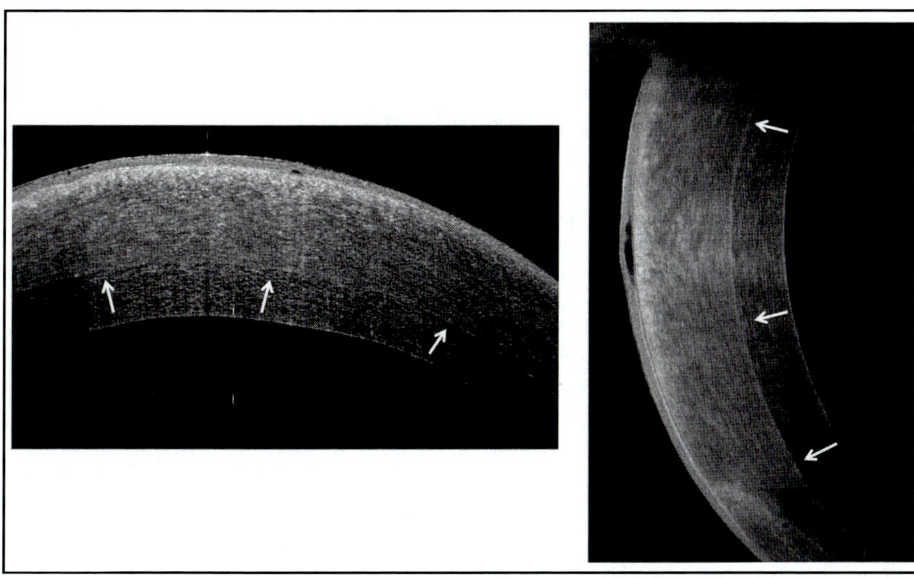

Figure 1-3. Anterior segment optical coherence tomography (OCT) showing pre-Descemetic DALK. Interface between host stroma and transplanted graft is seen (arrows).

ALK has several advantages over PK in that donor corneal requirements are not as stringent as for PK,[10] endothelial graft rejection is eliminated,[11] suture removal and discontinuation of topical steroids can be done earlier, and it also avoids the complications of an intraocular procedure.[12] Comparing PK with modern ALK did not

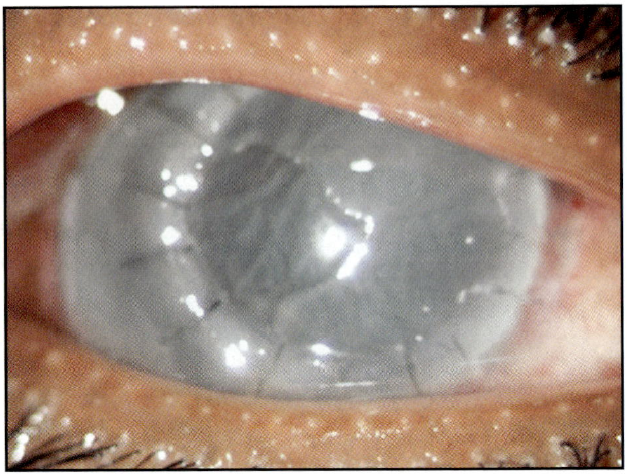

Figure 1-4. Persistent epithelial defect and interface haze in DALK.

see much difference with respect to postoperative refractive error and best-corrected visual acuity if residual stromal bed is minimal, but intraoperative complications like DM perforation forcing a conversion to PK, incomplete or irregular dissection, increased surgical time due to technical challenges, and postoperative complications, like interface haze (Figure 1-4), interface neovascularization, and pupillary block are some of the complications associated with LK.[12]

Posterior Lamellar Keratoplasty

Posterior lamellar keratoplasty involves replacing the host endothelium with healthy donor tissue in patients affected by Fuchs endothelial dystrophy and aphakic or pseudophakic bullous keratopathy.

Early History of Lamellar Keratoplasty

The German professor Arthur Von Hippel (1841–1916) advocated lamellar xenografts as far back as the end of the 19th century.[1] In 1877, Von Hippel used a trephine to prepare a human donor corneal graft of the same size and shape as the defect in the recipient cornea, which was left sutureless and kept in place only by pressure of the eyelids.[13] Eleven years later, von Hippel presented his new technique of circumscribed lamellar keratoplasty where he replaced a partial-thickness disc of the host's leucomatous cornea with a full-thickness xenograft from a dog. Von Hippel claimed that this technique was easier to perform than full-thickness keratoplasty and that complications of vitreous loss and displacement of other intraocular structures, such as the lens, was less when compared to full-thickness procedures resulted in complete healing at the end of 3 weeks with improvement in vision.[13] His outstanding experimental and clinical work showed that corneal endothelium and DM should remain intact if a corneal graft is to succeed.[14] Experiments in which partial thickness of the cornea was removed with a clockwork mechanical trephine and replaced with a full-thickness donor graft were attempted with good results as far back as the late 19th century.

In 1892, Fuchs reported on 30 lamellar grafts from rabbit, dog, and human eyes with disappointing results.[15]

Further modifications of lamellar keratoplasty was published in 1908 by Plange, who inserted oval full-thickness corneal grafts, like the face of a watch, into a corneal stromal pocket, and in 1910 by Lohlein, who used conjunctival flaps of the donor for securing a full-thickness corneal transplant.[13]

The mid-20th century saw a revival of lamellar keratoplasty with better clinical results from many corneal surgeons from around the world, including Barraquer in Columbia, Arruga in Spain, Rycroft in England, and Francheschetti in Switzerland.[16]

LK has evolved over time with attempts to achieve precision of depth and smoothness of both donor and recipient tissue to facilitate a smooth interface and optimize visual outcomes with the help of automation and sophisticated microsurgical instruments. The technical difficulties of LK and the suboptimal visual outcomes when compared to PK have led to numerous innovations in technique to overcome these drawbacks.

Lamellar corneal surgeries have undergone considerable evolution from the initial surgical attempts and the history of anterior and posterior LKs will be discussed separately.

Anterior Lamellar Keratoplasties

Initial attempts at LK toward the end of the 19th and beginning of the 20th century did not see much progress in the next 50 years due to the technical difficulties and interface haze of LK. The mid-20th century saw a resurgence in interest in LK with several innovations in LK giving better results. Peripheral lamellar grafts, large diameter grafts, and free-hand deep lamellar corneal dissection were attempted.[16]

Brown, while performing a PK in 1965, found it was possible to do deep dissection up to the DM leaving only bare DM and endothelium.[17] Baring of the DM provides a near perfect optical surface, but corneal surgeons of that period, including Anwar, felt that free hand dissection up to the DM was challenging, requiring a dry field and an operating microscope.[18]

The introduction of the microkeratome by Barraquer in 1964 to perform mechanical lamellar dissection of the cornea led to renewal in interest in lamellar procedures.[19]

Deep Anterior Lamellar Keratoplasty

DALK, the term coined for the surgical procedure in which the DM is bared, was first described by Sugita and Kondo[20] and has undergone numerous innovations in technique, including the use of air, fluid, or viscoelastic into the stromal layers to facilitate dissection

Direct Open Dissection (1974)

Anwar[21] used a partial-thickness trephine of 60% to 80% depth of the cornea after which the corneal stroma was removed in layers that became progressively more difficult as the DM was approached. This technically challenging procedure can still be used for patients with deep stromal scarring or inadequate visualization.

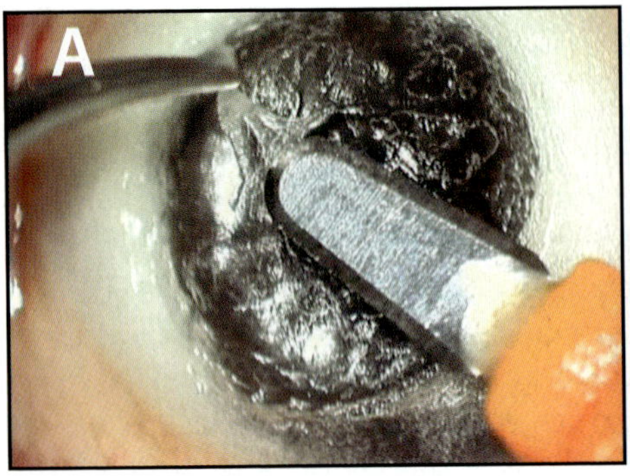

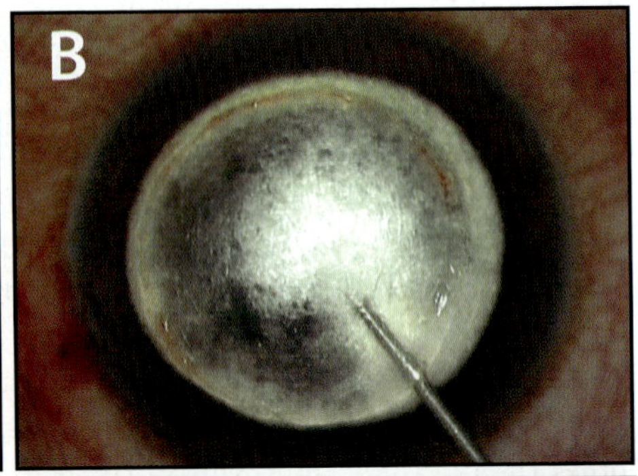

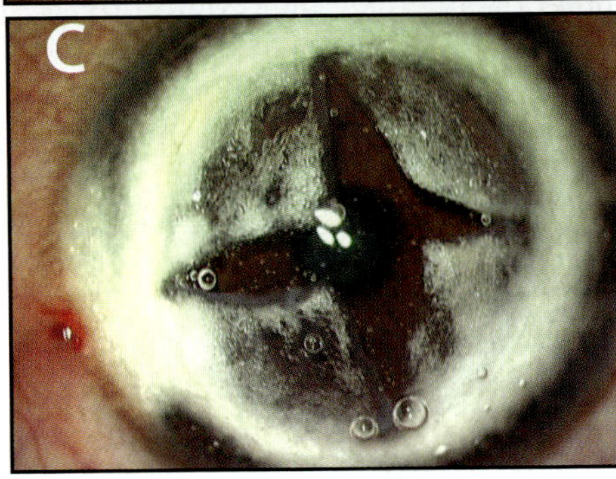

Figure 1-5. (A) Closed dissection using air in the anterior chamber as a guide (Melles technique). (B) Anwar's big bubble technique. (C) Four quadrant dissection. (Reprinted with permission from Dr. Soosan Jacob, Dr. Agarwal's Eye Hospital, Chennai, India.)

Intrastromal Air Injection (1985)

Intrastromal air injection[22] involves injection of air into the stroma after trephination to render it opaque and facilitate identification of the DM, which appears as a dark area, after which the stroma above is dissected with a spatula.

Dissection With Hydrodelamination

Saline is injected into the stromal bed after partial-thickness trephination, which whitens and swells and helps in the lamellar dissection of the stroma until the shiny smooth appearance of the DM is recognized.[20]

Dissection With Viscoelastics

Manche et al[23] and Melles et al[24] described dissection of the stromal layers using viscoelastics that were injected into a stromal pocket to help separate the DM from the stroma.

Closed Dissection

Replacement of the aqueous from the anterior chamber with air creating a mirror like air endothelium interface helped judge corneal depth so that a specially designed spatula could create a long deep stromal pocket over which the stroma was excised using a suction pocket (Figure 1-5A).[25]

Anwar's Big Bubble Technique (2002)

Big bubble technique described by Anwar and Teichmann is a faster, more reliable method of exposing the DM.[26] After the cornea is trephined up to 60% to 80%

depth with a suction trephine, a bent 27/30G needle with bevel down attached to an air-filled syringe is inserted deep into the stroma through the trephination groove, following which air is then injected deep into the stroma leading to the formation of a big bubble that spreads centrifugally in all directions. The big bubble detaches the central DM from the deeper stromal layers, helping in easier stromal dissection, following which a nick is made anterior to the big bubble through the remaining corneal layers. Remaining host stroma is divided into 4 quadrants and removed manually with blunt-tipped scissors (Figures 1-5B and 1-5C).

Big Bubble With Zigzag Femtosecond Laser

Big bubble combined with zigzag femtosecond laser for stromal dissection combines the advantages of minimizing postoperative astigmatism with the femto and the high-quality interface of the big bubble.[27]

Microkeratome-Assisted Lamellar Keratoplasty

Microkeratomes used for LASIK have been tried for stromal dissection in lamellar keratoplasties with microkeratomes helping in providing better precision, consistency, and optically smooth interfaces when compared to manual dissections.[28] It can be used for disorders affecting the anterior 250 μm of the cornea but can also be used for deeper pathology as long as sufficient stromal bed is available for structural integrity. Automated lamellar therapeutic keratoplasty uses the microkeratome for both recipient and donor lamellar dissection, ensuring perfect match between the recipient and donor, resulting in better visual outcomes.[29]

Automated lamellar therapeutic keratoplasties are continuously evolving in order to provide the best visual results and techniques that are not as challenging and difficult to do as the earlier procedures.

References

1. Moffatt SL, Cartwright VA, Stumpf TH. Centennial review of corneal transplantation. *Clin Exp Ophthalmol.* 2005;33(6):642-657. doi: 10.1111/j.1442-9071.2005.01134.x
2. Pellier de Quengsy G. *Précis Ou Cours D'opérations Sur La Chirurgie Des Yeux ... Par M.G. Pellier de Quengsy, Fils.* Paris, France: Didot; 1789.
3. Bigger SLL. An inquiry into the possibility of transplanting the cornea, with the view of relieving blindness (hitherto deemed incurable) caused by several diseases of that structure. *Dublin J Med Sci.* 1837;11(3):408-417.
4. Kissam R. Ceratoplastics in man. *New York J Med.* 1844;2:281-282.
5. Zirm E. Eine erfolgreiche totale Keratoplastik. *Albr von Græfe's Arch für Ophthalmol.* 1906;64(3):580-593.
6. Filatov VP. Transplantation of the cornea from preserved cadavers' eyes. *Lancet.* 1937;229(5937):1395-1397.
7. Krumeich JH, Schoner P, Lubatschowski H, Gerten G, Kermani O. [Excimer laser treatment in deep lamellar keratoplasty 100 micrometer over Descemet's membrane]. *Ophthalmologe.* 2002;99(12):946-948. doi: 10.1007/s00347-002-0670-5
8. Hafezi F, Mrochen M, Fankhauser F II, Seiler T. Anterior lamellar keratoplasty with a microkeratome: a method for managing complications after refractive surgery. *J Refract Surg.* 2003;19(1):52-57.
9. Price FW Jr. Air lamellar keratoplasty. *Refract Corneal Surg.* 1989;5:240-243.

10. Shimazaki J. The evolution of lamellar keratoplasty. *Curr Opin Ophthalmol.* 2000;11(4):217-223. doi: 10.1097/00055735-200008000-00002
11. Terry MA. The evolution of lamellar grafting techniques over twenty-five years. *Cornea.* 2000;19(5):611-616. doi: 10.1097/00003226-200009000-00006
12. Reinhart WJ, Musch DC, Jacobs DS, Lee WB, Kaufman SC, Shtein RM. Deep anterior lamellar keratoplasty as an alternative to penetrating keratoplasty: a report by the American Academy of Ophthalmology. *Ophthalmology.* 2011;118(1):209-218. doi: 10.1016/j.ophtha.2010.11.002
13. Forrester JV. *Corneal Transplantation.* London, United Kingdom: Imperial College Press; 2004.
14. von Graefe A. Albrecht von Graefe and glaucoma. *Arch Ophthalmol.* 1888;34:108.
15. Trevor Roper PD. *The History of Corneal Grafting.* London, United Kingdom: Butterworth; 1972.
16. Arenas E, Esquenazi S, Anwar M, Terry M. Lamellar corneal transplantation. *Surv Ophthalmol.* 2012;57(6):510-529. doi: 10.1016/j.survophthal.2012.01.009
17. Brown SL, Dohlman CH. Dislocation of Descemet's membrane during keratoplasty. *Am J Ophthalmol.* 1965;60:43-45.
18. Anwar M. Planned near-Descemet's dissection in deep lamellar keratoplasty, using air and fluid. In: John T, ed. *Surgical Techniques in Anterior and Posterior Lamellar Corneal Surgery.* New Delhi, India: Jaypee Brothers; 2006:126-133.
19. JI B. Queratomileusis para la correccion de la miopia. *Arch Soc Am Oftalmol Optom.* 1964;5:27-28.
20. Sugita J, Kondo J. Deep lamellar keratoplasty with complete removal of pathological stroma for vision improvement. *Br J Ophthalmol.* 1997;81(3):184. doi: 10.1136/bjo.81.3.184
21. Anwar M. Dissection technique in lamellar keratoplasty. *Br J Ophthalmol.* 1972;56(9):711-713.
22. Archila EA. Deep lamellar keratoplasty dissection of host tissue with intrastromal air injection. *Cornea.* 1984;3(3):217-218.
23. Manche EE, Holland GN, Maloney RK. Deep lamellar keratoplasty using viscoelastic dissection. *Arch Ophthalmol.* 1999;117(11):1561-1565. doi: 10.1001/archopht.117.11.1561
24. Melles GR, Remeijer L, Geerards AJ, Beekhuis WH. A quick surgical technique for deep, anterior lamellar keratoplasty using visco-dissection. *Cornea.* 2000;19(4):427-432. doi: 10.1097/00003226-200007000-00004
25. Melles GR, Rietveld FJ, Beekhuis WH, Binder PS. A technique to visualize corneal incision and lamellar dissection depth during surgery. *Cornea.* 1999;18(1):80-86. doi: 00003226-199901000-00013
26. Anwar M. Technique in lamellar keratoplasty. *Trans Ophthalmol Soc UK.* 1974;94:163-171.
27. Suwan-Apichon O, Reyes JMG, Griffin NB, Barker J, Gore P, Chuck RS. Microkeratome versus femtosecond laser predissection of corneal grafts for anterior and posterior lamellar keratoplasty. *Cornea.* 2006;25(8):966-968. doi: 10.1097/01.ico.0000226360.34301.29
28. Azar DT. A new surgical technique of microkeratome-assisted deep lamellar keratoplasty with a hinged flap. *Arch Ophthalmol.* 2000;118(8):1112.
29. Tan DTH, Mehta JS. Future directions in lamellar corneal transplantation. *Cornea.* 2007;26(9 suppl 1):S21-8. doi: 10.1097/ICO.0b013e31812f685c

Please see videos on the accompanying website at
www.healio.com/books/DALKvideos

2

Anterior Lamellar Versus Penetrating Keratoplasty

Leopoldo Spadea, MD and Vittoria De Rosa, MD

The purpose of corneal transplantation[1-59] is to replace the pathological cornea of the eye with a normal clear cornea. In penetrating keratoplasty (PK) the full thickness of the cornea is replaced, while in anterior lamellar keratoplasty (ALK) the corneal stroma is replaced down to the Descemet's membrane (DM), so that the healthy endothelium of the recipient is left intact. Although the desired therapeutic outcomes of the 2 procedures are identical with respect to restoring vision and biomechanical efficiency, the benefits and the risk profile may be different. Replacing fewer layers of the cornea may reduce the likelihood of rejection and subsequent failure because the endothelium is retained.

Contemporary corneal transplantation techniques are the result of years of ideas, experimentations, and perseverance over centuries. PK, a procedure involving the replacement of a full-thickness portion of the cornea, has been the dominant surgical approach for most causes of corneal blindness for more than half a century. The first successful human corneal graft dates back to 1905 when the Austrian Eduard Zirm transplanted a full-thickness human cornea from an 11-year-old boy onto a woman's eye, restoring her vision.[1] Starting from the Zirm's success, with the development of corticosteroids, antibiotics, surgical microscopes, and improved trephines, several physicians have contributed to the refinement of corneal transplantation, making PK the treatment of choice for corneal diseases.[2] In recent years, however, the concept of lamellar keratoplasty (LK) has emerged, leading to a fundamental change in the history of corneal transplantation. This technique aims to selectively replace the diseased corneal stroma without removing the DM and endothelium so as to minimize unnecessary replacement of the unaffected healthy layer. As mentioned earlier, by

Jacob S, ed. *Mastering DALK: A Video Textbook on Deep Anterior Lamellar Keratoplasty* (pp 9-25).

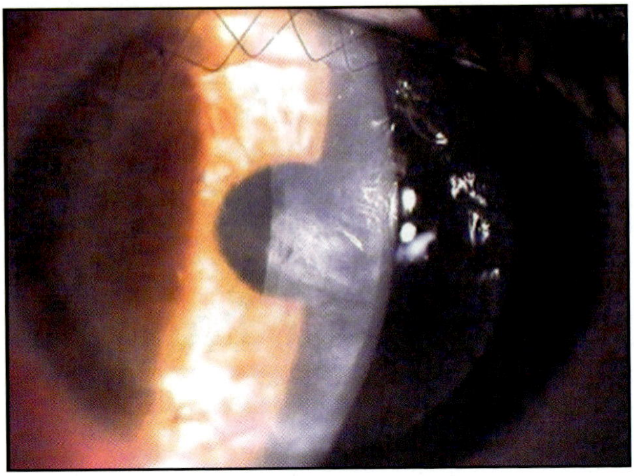

Figure 2-1. Biomicroscopic examination 3 months after pre-Descemetic DALK (PD-DALK) in a 29-year old keratoconus patient. Opacity and folds in the interface between donor and recipient cornea are visible.

retaining the patient's own endothelium, the risk of endothelial rejection, a major cause of graft failure in PK, is almost eliminated and endothelial cell density is preserved. Consequently, there is no need for long-term immunosuppressive therapy with corticosteroids, decreasing the risk of cataract, glaucoma, and infections.[3]

With the aid of new surgical devices, such as advanced microkeratome instrumentation, excimer laser, and femtosecond laser, several authors have ventured into LK surgery utilizing different techniques. All their efforts are aimed at creating a smooth interface between host and donor tissues, thus reducing refractive irregularities.

In this regard, the field of the ALK can be divided into 2 main categories: ALK with augmented thickness and deep anterior lamellar keratoplasty (DALK). The first one includes all those techniques aimed at achieving both a thickening and a reshaping of the cornea by using a thick donor lamella of normal curvature[4-8]; the second one consists of techniques in which the dissection of the host tissue is close to the DM, so that a smooth and transparent recipient bed is achieved.[9,10]

Some surgeons believe that leaving in place a small portion of posterior stroma, without completely baring the DM, prevents microperforations from becoming macroperforations, thus providing better results. This is why they prefer to PD-DALK when LK enables the removal of three-quarters or more of stroma to the deeper layers[11] (Figures 2-1 through 2-3). On the other hand, there are those who are convinced that the surgery outcome depends on the creation of a cleavage plane as deep as possible, so that in the last decade several techniques of maximum depth dissection have been proposed[12,13] (Figure 2-4). Among these, the most successful is certainly the *big bubble technique*, first introduced by Anwar in 2002.[14] Several variations of this technique have been proposed over the years, including hydrodissection, viscodissection, and manual dissection,[15,16] that are performed by worldwide experts with encouraging results.[17-21]

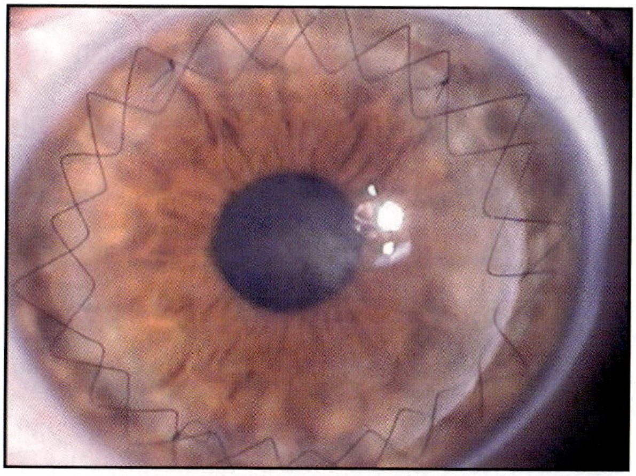

Figure 2-2. Clinical appearance 6 months postoperatively of a PD-DALK. Two double running 10-0 nylon suture are visible. The opacity in the interface is less visible.

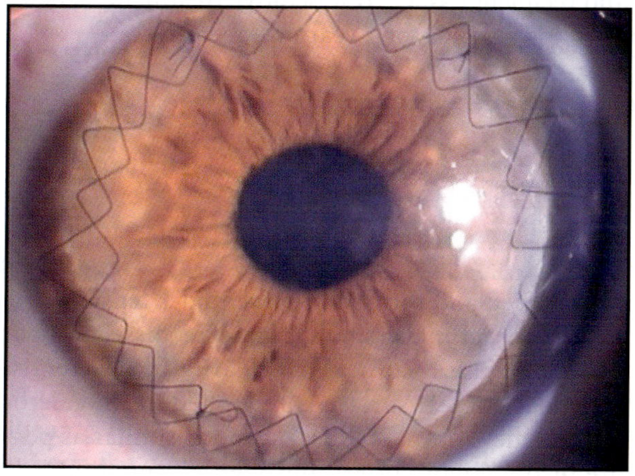

Figure 2-3. Slit lamp appearance of a PD-DALK 1 year postoperatively. The graft is clear and the interface barely visible. The cloudiness has quite disappeared.

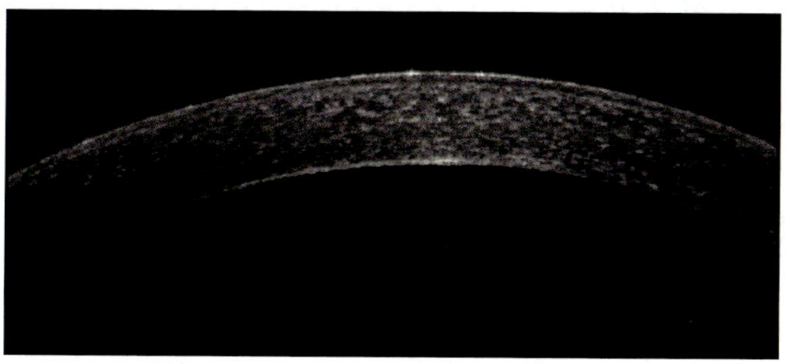

Figure 2-4. Optical coherence tomography (OCT) images of a patient after DALK. A healthy epithelium and the interface between donor and recipient cornea are notable.

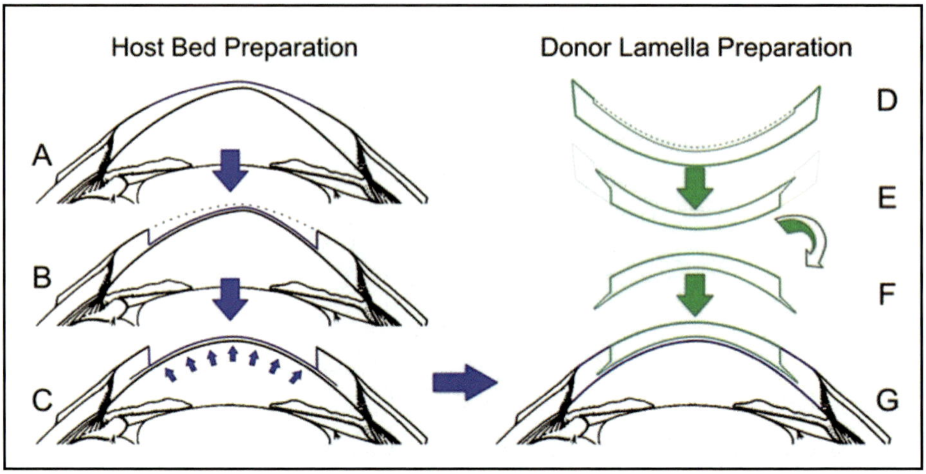

Figure 2-7. CLAT technique. (A) The recipient cornea (B) is prepared to remove the irregular keratoconic thickness by custom excimer laser ablation, (C) resulting in the formation of a uniform thickness receiving bed. (D) The laser first thins the donor cornea (E) and then shapes the donor perimeter to create a saddle and obtain a wing of the lamella. After it is punched, (F) the completed donor, as a complement to the planned recipient bed, (G) is sutured in place, yielding a full-thickness normalized postoperative condition.

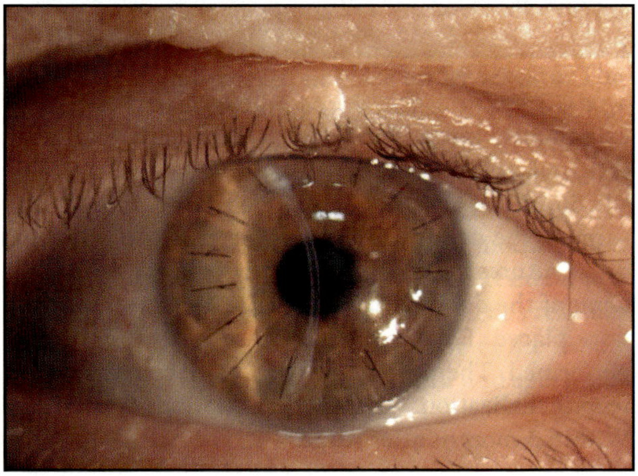

Figure 2-8. Biomicroscopic examination. Lamellar graft in a 21-year-old keratoconus patient 2 weeks after CLAT for keratoconus. Sixteen interrupted 10-0 nylon sutures are visible.

a suction punch. The receiving bed is created using a 3-dimensional pachymetry map obtained from the tomographer and calculating the intersection of an ideal surface referenced from the posterior surface of the cornea. The irregular volume above this ideal surface is ablated with excimer laser. Using a circular movement with a disc knife a 2.0-mm stromal pocket is obtained around the circumference of the ablation floor. The donor lamella is then secured into the recipient bed with 4 cardinal sutures and the wing of the donor lamella is introduced into the stromal pocket and 16 interrupted 10-0 nylon sutures are finally placed[24] (Figures 2-7 through 2-10 and Video 2-1).

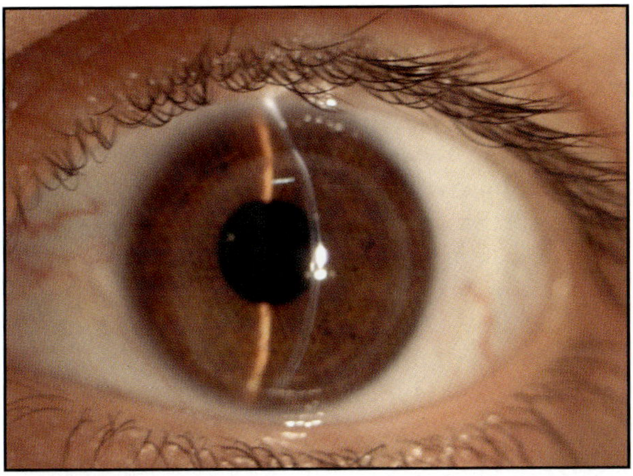

Figure 2-9. Two years after CLAT, the graft appears clear with no interface scarring.

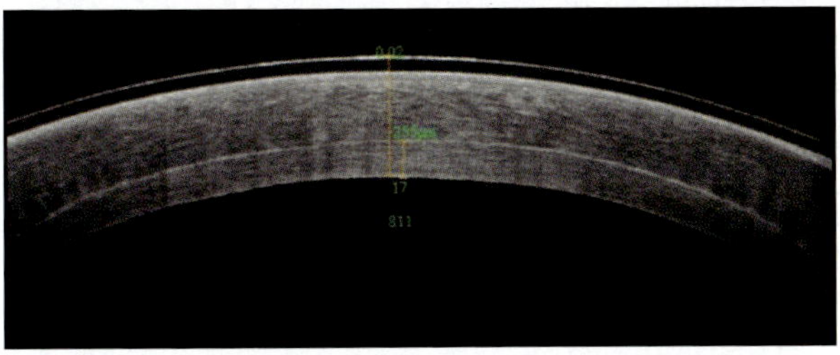

Figure 2-10. OCT image showing the perfect match between donor and recipient tissues 7 days after CLAT. A soft bandage contact lens is visible.

Femtosecond Laser–Assisted Lamellar Keratoplasty

The capability of the femtosecond laser to photodisrupt tissue with minimal collateral damage has made it a promising tool for increasing accuracy and predictability in corneal surgery. The laser is used to prepare both the donor lamella and the recipient bed. Because the laser pulses result in multiple corneal intrastromal gas bubbles (ie, microcavitations), it requires only a manual light lamellar dissection with a blunted spatula to create the intrastromal cut with a smooth surface. After the procedure, the donor lamella is secured in the recipient bed with 10-0 nylon sutures. At the end of surgery, a soft contact lens is placed on the eye surface to assist epithelial healing.

It has been claimed that the reproducibility of the lamellar cuts in the donor and recipient corneas provided by the femtosecond laser may decrease the necessity of corneal suturing, thus allowing for an early visual rehabilitation.[25]

DALK

Among DALK techniques, the most performed is certainly the big bubble technique. It consists of a partial trephination of the cornea, performed with a calibrated guided trephine, to a depth between 60% and 80%. A 27- or 30-gauge needle attached to an air-filled syringe is inserted into the deep stroma through the bottom of the trephination groove and a forceful injection of air causes the separation of the DM from the corneal stroma. The bubble appears as a circular area with a dense white border corresponding to the trephination groove. A keratectomy, anterior to the big bubble, is carefully performed so as not to accidentally breech the bubble. Then the bubble is pierced near the center of the cornea and an opening in the anterior wall of the air-pocket is formed. Viscoelastic is injected and scissors are used to divide the anterior stroma into 4 sections, which are then removed exposing the DM, by cutting each quadrant at the edge of the trephination. The detection of a sixth layer of the cornea, the Dua's layer, beyond the last row of kerotocytes, led the surgeon to assume that the big bubble cleaves off a distinct layer at the posterior surface of the corneal stroma, which is not residual stroma but a well-defined, acellular strong layer.[26] For the preparation of the donor cornea the lamella is punched out from the endothelium side and the DM with endothelium is gently stripped off with a dry sponge. Then the button is sutured in place using two continuous, 12-bite, 10-0 nylon sutures or 24 interrupted sutures (Figures 2-11 and 2-12 and Video 2-2).

Sugita and Kondo[27] described the *hydrodelamination technique*, a procedure combining air and fluid injection. A saline solution is injected in a small depression, which is created in the deeper stroma after a partial trephination. This procedure helps to achieve a cleavage plane over DM so that the loosened tissue can be removed in thin layers with forceps and scissors. The DM is recognized from its shiny and smooth appearance.

Farid and Steinert[28] introduced a new approach combining big bubble DALK with the femtosecond laser zigzag incision in which the matching and interlocking donor-host wound increases surface area and create a customized donor-host match. In a zigzag incision, the laser creates an angled posterior cut, a lamellar ring cut in mid-stroma, and an angled anterior cut, each of which intersect. According to Farid and Steinert,[28] this type of wound allows rapid healing and good biomechanical stability. Furthermore, the laser cut allows an exact cut depth within 70 μm of the DM, allowing more precise placement of the air needle.

Yao[15], in an attempt to achieve a thorough removal of the stroma, developed the hooking detaching technique. It consists of creating a pocket in the recipient bed by means of a three-quarter trephination, followed by a peeling of the remnant stroma to approach DM along the trephined margin in the area between 11 and 1 o'clock by the aid of a golf-shaped knife. In this area the residual stromal fibers are hooked and lifted by forceps with a tip of concaved teeth for the consequent exposure of the DM. A 27-gauge cannula connected to a syringe containing viscoelastic is inserted in the pocket between the stroma and the DM and the injection of viscoelastic material allows the detachment process.[15]

A research line other than the techniques described up to now was disclosed by Tsubota et al in 1998.[29] Tsubota's divide-and-conquer technique differs from the others because the DM deep dissection is not performed by injecting any substances and it is practiced completely manually. It originally derives from the application of cataract phacoemulsification technique to the deep lamellar keratoplasty. The corneal stroma is divided into 4 quadrants to facilitate lamellar dissection at approximately

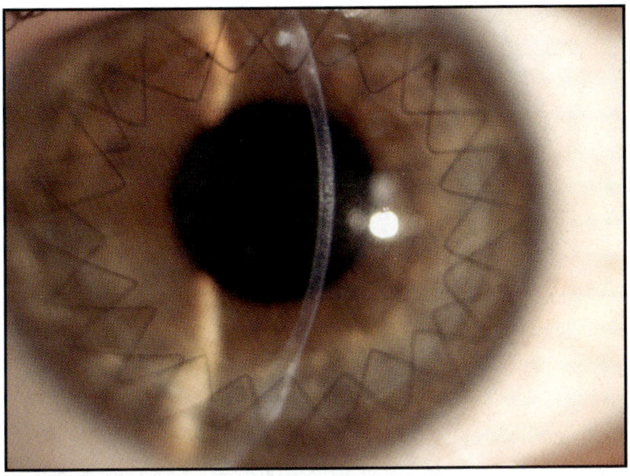

Figure 2-11. Biomicroscopic examination showed a clear and well-integrated lamellar graft in a 35-year-old keratoconus patient who had Descemetic DALK (big bubble technique) 6 months previously. Two double-running 12-bite sutures are present.

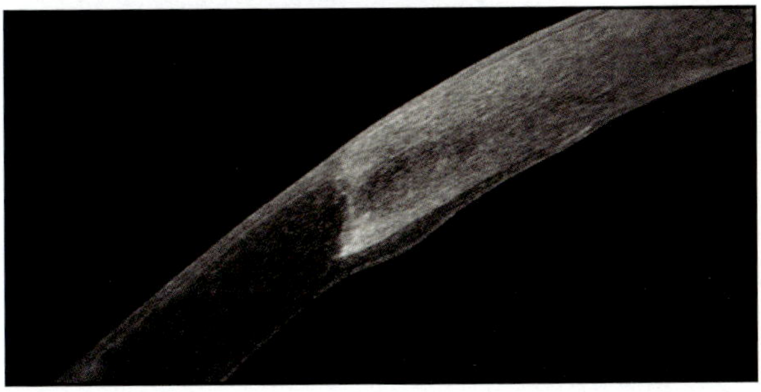

Figure 2-12. Anterior segment Fourier-domain OCT image 2 years after DALK. Note the edge of the lamellar graft firmly included in the host cornea.

70% deep, until the DM is exposed in the central area. In this way it increases the repeatability and the standardization of the procedure.

Comparison of Penetrating Keratoplasty and Anterior Lamellar Keratoplasty: Risks and Benefits Analysis

There are plenty of studies in the literature comparing the outcomes of ALK and PK[3,30,31] (Tables 2-1 and 2-2). The American Academy of Ophthalmology recommends DALK as a preferred technique.[32] Graft failure remains the main problem of PK surgery because it has a rate of incidence that ranges from 18% to 34% (Figure 2-13). The major reason for graft failure is endothelial rejection, which occurs in more than 50% of all the cases. A large cohort study with a 15-year follow-up showed that the endothelial cell density continues to decrease after PK, until it stabilizes approximately 10 years after surgery, when the total endothelial cell loss is estimated to be around 70% compared to presurgical values.[33] Felipe et al,[34] in a study on 149 eyes of 109 patients submitted to PK, with the most common indication of keratoconus (76.5%), with a

Table 2-1

Advantages and Disadvantages of Penetrating Keratoplasty and Anterior Lamellar Keratoplasty

	Penetrating Keratoplasty	Anterior Lamellar Keratoplasty
Advantages	• Dominant procedure for half a century • Different set of intraoperative complications, sometimes vision threatening • Shorter learning curve	• Lower endothelial cell loss rate • Lower risk of endothelial rejection and graft failure • No need for long-term immunosuppressive therapy • Earlier suture removal • Faster visual recovery
Disadvantages	• Open-eye surgery • Higher endothelial cell loss rate • Higher incidence of endothelial rejection and graft failure • Long-term immunosuppressive therapy needs • Higher risk of cataract and glaucoma • Delayed visual recovery	• Steeper surgical learning curve • Technically more difficult and time-consuming surgery until mastered • Higher intraoperative complication rate, though generally not sight threatening • Possible refractive irregularities at the donor/host junction

follow-up of at least 20 years or more, evidenced postoperative complications including rejection (29.5%), cataract formation (26.2%), and steroid-induced elevated intraocular pressure (15.4%). Moreover, peripheral thinning and ectasia diagnosed by slit lamp were noted in 59 eyes (39.6%), most of which were mild (54.2%), inferiorly located (66.1%), and involved the graft-host junction (81.4%). Most of the grafts that developed ectasia had a preoperative diagnosis of keratoconus (91.5%) (Figure 2-14).

On the contrary, the major advantage of ALK vs PK is the low rate of endothelial cell loss and graft rejection, because the patient's own endothelium is retained; however, this technique is more time-consuming, technically demanding, and dependent on the surgeons' skill than PK.[15] Despite this fact, however, it is still logical to

Table 2-2

Outcomes and Complication Rates Among the Different Techniques

	PK [22,51-53]	DALK [9,12,17-19]	Microkeratome LK [5-8]	Excimer Laser LK [4,23-24,54]	Femtosecond Laser LK [55-57]
Mean CDVA	0.63 ± 0.19	0.74 ± 0.11	0.63 ± 0.12	0.68 ± 0.08	0.44 ± 0.19
Mean RA	2.61 ± 0.64	2.62 ± 0.29	3.64 ± 0.65	1.77 ± 0.66	3.32 ± 0.36
Graft Failure %	22.67 ± 20.33	6.32 ± 5.69	0	0	4.76 ± 8.24
Postoperative High IOP %	6.34 ± 6.34	4.66 ± 10.24	0	0	9.52 ± 16.49
Cataract %	2.94 ± 2.90	2.27 ± 4.16	0.005 ± 0.01	0	0

CDVA = corrected distance visual acuity; IOP = intraocular pressure; RA = refractive astigmatism.

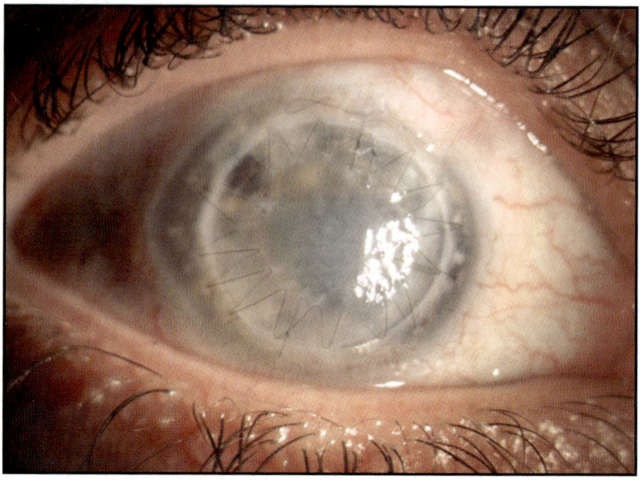

Figure 2-13. Biomicroscopic examination 14 months after PK. Noticeable corneal edema and folds in the recipient cornea are visible.

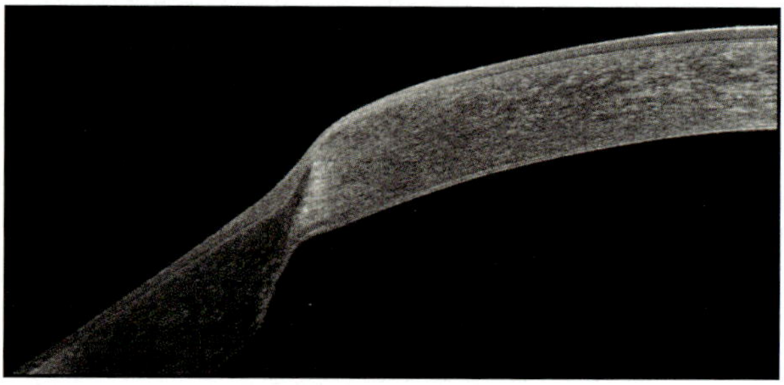

Figure 2-14. ASOCT image showing peripheral thinning and ectasia with segment elevation between donor and recipient cornea 18 years after PK.

primarily attempt an ALK surgery in keratoconic patients and thereby have to convert to a PK only in those cases where an irretrievable complication occurs.

In MALK, potential complications include lack of precision in flap diameter obtained in both recipient and donor dissection (because flap diameter is in part dependent on the variable suction pressures), epithelial ingrowths in the interface, delays or defects in epithelialization, fibrosis, and even vascularization.[5-8]

The femtosecond laser uses a type of near-infrared light with a wavelength of 1053 nm that is able to perform bladeless, precise, and predefined lamellar cuts with minimal tissue injury. The femtosecond laser presents a cutting accuracy twice as high compared to the mechanical microkeratome.[25,35-37] However, complications, such as mild interface haze, interface inflammation, recurrence of pathology, and dry eye, are not uncommon.

The excimer laser offers the advantage of enabling a custom ablation for both the receiving bed and the lamella. It means that it is possible to plan different ablation depths in the same cornea as a function of corneal thickness differentials. It also seems to be a safe and more standardized procedure, but long surgical times and high levels of laser energy, with possible risk of endothelium damage, are needed.[4,23-24]

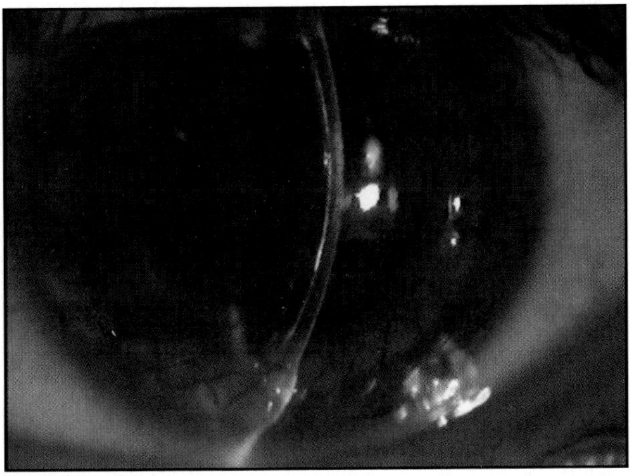

Figure 2-15. Slit lamp appearance 7 days after DALK. Double-chamber formation is evident.

The most feared complication of DALK surgery is inadvertent DM perforation, which has a rate of incidence between 2.3% and 32%.[38] A limbal paracentesis, with the aim of lowering the intraocular pressure, helps to decrease the risk of perforation[39]; however, in the majority of the cases, it is often possible to continue DALK surgery. Irretrievable large perforations can be managed with a conversion to PK, with satisfactory results.[40] Another possible complication of DALK is the formation of a double anterior chamber during the intrastromal air injection, due to the fact that the needle is not advanced deep enough into the posterior stromal layer[41] (Figure 2-15). Furthermore, the visual acuity after surgery could be reduced by central folds in the DM. A mismatch between the recipient bed size and the donor button is responsible for folds. Oversizing the donor button by 0.25 to 0.5 mm can help prevent this complication, while same size button can help decrease large myopic refractive errors if any.

Other complications, such as pupillary blockage from mismanagement of the air bubble in the anterior chamber or a fixed dilated pupil (ie, Urrets-Zavalia syndrome), may occur when an inexperienced surgeon performs ALK.[42]

Although refractive outcomes of lamellar surgery have been promoted as being significantly better than that of the well-established alternative of PK,[43,44] various reports differ with respect to evidence for this claim. Keane et al[45] stated that there are no differences between DALK and PK in terms of best-corrected visual acuity (BCVA), spherical equivalent, and keratometric astigmatism in patients with keratoconus. In their review, Reinhart et al[46] concluded that the 2 techniques lead to equivalent BCVA and refractive outcomes. Shi et al[47] found out that PK led to greater improvement in BCVA, no differences in refractive outcomes, and less rejection with DALK. The review by Henein and Nanavaty,[48] on the other hand, showed strong evidence of better postoperative refractive astigmatism following DALK but no difference in spherical equivalent or keratometric astigmatism between DALK and PK.

Moreover, while it is true that DALK eliminates the risk of endothelial rejection, it is also true that stromal and epithelial rejections are similar between DALK and

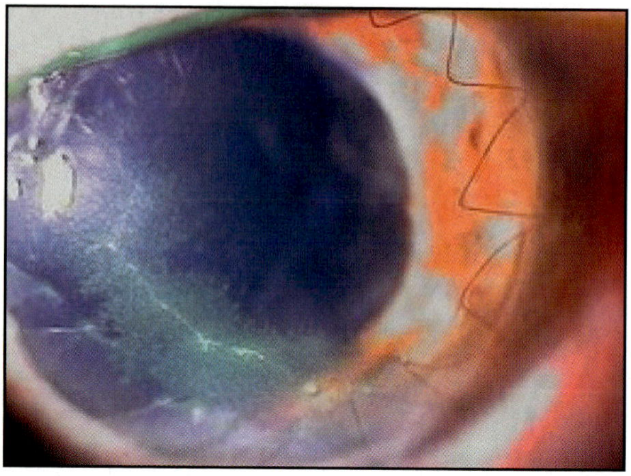

Figure 2-16. Biomicroscopic examination 12 months after PK. An evident epithelial rejection in the donor cornea is visible. Epithelial rejection may also be seen after DALK but generally recovers rapidly.

PK (Figure 2-16). However, epithelial rejection is usually mild and can be attenuated quickly by topical steroids.[49] Furthermore, because DALK is an extraocular procedure, it lacks the risk associated with open-eye surgery, such as iris/lens damage, expulsive hemorrhage, and endophthalmitis. In addition, sutures can be removed earlier, which is beneficial to postoperative rehabilitation.[50] Nevertheless loose sutures may be more common among DALK patients than PK patients, probably due to the fact that, because the surgeon is aware of the risk of perforating the DM if the needle is passed very deep during suturing, sutures could be inadvertently placed superficially.[50]

Abdelkader,[51] in his work, discusses clinical outcome of DALK and PK with emphasis on corneal biomechanics and wound healing. He states that in DALK the wound healing comes from 2 sources: the deep lamellar interface and the peripheral wound edge, while in PK the healing comes only from the wound edge. The healing area in DALK is therefore more extensive. This combined healing after DALK contributes to the adherence and the integrity of the graft inducing superior wound strength and hence better corneal biomechanics in the early postoperative period. Other authors before him attributed the better corneal biomechanics in DALK eyes to the only intactness of DM in these eyes; however, at 1 year the corneal biomechanics of DALK and PK seems to be comparable.

Lastly, something more we have to take into account is that DALK also offers fewer rigid criteria for donor graft selection as viable donor endothelium is not required. This is particularly important in countries where donor tissues are exiguous.[52]

Conclusion

Benefits and risk profiles of the 2 procedures are different. Replacing fewer layers of the cornea may reduce the likelihood of rejection and subsequent failure, but other complications similar to that of PK may arise due to problems at the donor/host junction. Since the introduction of DALK, there has been progressive improvement in visual outcomes due to improved surgical techniques and surgeons' experience. Furthermore, DALK can be performed with donor tissue that would not be suitable for PK because of inadequate endothelial cell density, a factor that would substantially increase the availability of tissue suitable for corneal transplantation. Thus, the benefits of DALK outweigh the risk of additional complications and DALK should, therefore, be performed whenever appropriate.

References

1. Crawford AZ, Patel DV, McGhee CJN. A brief history of corneal transplantation: From ancient to modern. *Oman J Ophthalmol.* 2013;6(1):12-17
2. Pramanik S, Musch DC, Sutphin JE, Farjo AA. Extended long-term outcomes of penetrating keratoplasty for keratoconus. *Ophthalmology.* 2006;113:1633-1638.
3. Coster DJ, Lowe MT, Keane MC; Australian Corneal Graft Registry Contributors. A comparison of lamellar and penetrating keratoplasty outcomes: a registry study. *Ophthalmology.* 2014;121(5):978-987.
4. Buratto L, Belloni S, Valeri R. Excimer laser lamellar keratoplasty of augmented thickness for keratoconus. *J Refract Surg.* 1998;14(5):517-525.
5. Busin M, Zambianchi L, Arffa RC. Microkeratome-assisted lamellar keratoplasty for the surgical treatment of keratoconus. *Ophthalmology.* 2005;112(6):987-997.
6. Busin M, Scorcia V, Zambianchi L, Ponzin D. Outcomes from a modified microkeratome-assisted lamellar keratoplasty for keratoconus. *Arch Ophthalmol.* 2012;130(6):776-782.
7. Bilgihan K, Ozdek S, Sari A, Hasanreisoglu B. Microkeratome-assisted lamellar keratoplasty for keratoconus: stromal sandwich. *J Cataract Refract Surg.* 2003;29(7):1267-1272.
8. Acar BT, Arslan OS, Buttanri IB, Sevim MS, Acar S. Comparing deep anterior lamellar keratoplasty and automated lamellar therapeutic keratoplasty in patients with keratoconus. *Jpn J Ophthalmol.* 2011; 55(4):327-332.
9. Rama P, Knutsson KA, Razzoli G, Matuska S, Viganò M, Paganoni G. Deep anterior lamellar keratoplasty using an original manual technique. *Br J Ophthalmol.* 2013;97(1):23-27.
10. Marchini G, Mastropasqua L, Pedrotti E, et al. Deep lamellar keratoplasty by intracorneal dissection: a prospective clinical confocal microscopic study. *Ophthalmology.* 2006;113(8):1289-1300.
11. Sarnicola V, Toro P, Gentile D, Hannush SB. Descemetic DALK and predescemetic DALK: outcomes in 236 cases of keratoconus. *Cornea.* 2010;29(1):53-59.
12. MacIntyre R, Chow SP, Chan E, Poon A. Long-term outcomes of deep anterior lamellar keratoplasty versus penetrating keratoplasty in Australian keratoconus patients. *Cornea.* 2014;33(1):6-9.
13. Cano-Ortiz A, Villarrubia A. Corneal transplantation in keratoconus: penetrating keratoplasty versus deep anterior lamellar keratoplasty with Melles technique. *Arch Soc Esp Oftalmol.* 2015;90(1):4-8.
14. Anwar M, Teichmann KD. Big-bubble technique to bare Descemet's membrane in anterior lamellar keratoplasty. *J Cataract Refract Surg.* 2002;28(3):398-403.
15. Yao YF. A novel technique for performing full-bed deep lamellar keratoplasty. *Cornea.* 2008:27;19-24.
16. Farid M, Steinert RF. Deep anterior lamellar keratoplasty performed with the femtosecond laser zigzag incision for the treatment of stromal corneal pathology and ecstatic disease. *J Cataract Refract Surg.* 2009;35(5):809-813.
17. Romano V, Iovieno A, Parente G, Soldani AM, Fontana L. Long-term clinical outcomes of deep anterior lamellar keratoplasty in patients with keratoconus. *Am J Ophthalmol.* 2015;159(3):505-511.
18. Khakshoor H, Eslampoor A, Rad SS, Vejdani A. Modified deep anterior lamellar keratoplasty for the treatment of advanced keratoconus with steep corneal curvature to help in eliminating the wrinkles in the Descemet's membrane. *Indian J Ophthalmol.* 2014;62(4):392-395.

19. Fogla R, Padmanabhan P. Results of deep lamellar keratoplasty using the big-bubble technique in patients with keratoconus. *Am J Ophthalmol.* 2006;141:254-259.
20. Fontana L, Parente G, Tassinari G . Clinical outcomes after deep anterior lamellar keratoplasty using the big-bubble technique in patients with keratoconus. *Am J Ophthalmol.* 2007;143:117-124.
21. Al-Torbak AA, Al-Motowa S, Al-Assiri A, Al-Kharashi S, Al-Shahwan S, Al-Mezaine H. Deep anterior lamellar keratoplasty for keratoconus. *Cornea.* 2006;25:408-412.
22. Choi JA, Lee MA, Kim MS. Long-term outcomes of penetrating keratoplasty in keratoconus: analysis of the factors associated with final visual acuities. *Int J Ophthalmol.* 2014;7(3):517-21.
23. Spadea L, Giammaria D, Fascia A, Verrecchia V. Excimer laser-assisted lamellar keratoplasty for the treatment of keratoconus. *J Cataract Refract Surg.* 2009;35(1):105-112.
24. Spadea L, Gizzi R, Evangelista Conocchia N, Urbano S. Optical pachimetry–guided custom excimer laser-assisted lamellar keratoplasty for the surgical treatment of keratoconus. *J Cataract Refract Surg.* 2012;38(3):1559-1567.
25. Baradaran-Rafii A, Eslani M. Femtosecond laser assisted corneal transplantation. *Br J Ophthalmol.* 2013;97(6):675-676.
26. Dua HS, Faraj LA, Said DG, Gray T, Lowe J. Human corneal anatomy redefined: a novel pre-Descemet's layer (Dua's layer). *Ophthalmology.* 2013;120(9):1778-1785.
27. Sugita J, Kondo J. Deep lamellar keratoplasty with complete removal of pathological stroma for vision improvement. *Br J Ophthalmol.* 1997;81(3):184-188.
28. Farid M, Steinert RF. Deep anterior lamellar keratoplasty performed with the femtosecond laser zigzag incision for the treatment of stromal corneal pathology and ecstatic disease. *J Cataract Refract Surg.* 2009;35(5):809-813.
29. Tsubota K, Kaido M, Monden Y, Satake Y, Bissen-Miyajima H, Shimazaki J. A new surgical technique for deep lamellar keratoplasty with single running suture adjustment. *Am J Ophthalmol.* 1998;126(1):1-8.
30. Bahar I, Kaiserman I, Srinivasan S, Ya Ping J, Slomovic AR, Rootman DS. Comparison of three different techniques of corneal transplantation for keratoconus. *Am J Ophthalmol.* 2008;146:905-912.
31. Funnell CL, Ball J, Noble BA. Comparative cohort study of the outcomes of deep lamellar keratoplasty and penetrating keratoplasty for keratoconus. *Eye.* 2006;20:527-532.
32. Reinhart WJ, Musch DC, Jacobs DS, Lee WB, Kaufman SC, Shtein RM. Deep anterior lamellar keratoplasty as an alternative to penetrating keratoplasty a report by the American Academy of Ophthalmology. *Ophthalmology.* 2011;118(1):209-18.
33. Patel SV, Hodge DO, Bourne WM. Corneal endothelium and postoperative outcomes 15 years after penetrating keratoplasty. *Am J Ophthalmol.* 2005;139:311-319.
34. Felipe AF, Hammersmith KM, Nottage JM, Rapuano CJ, Nagra PK, Cohen EJ, Laibson PR. Indications, visual outcome, and ectasia in clear corneal transplants 20 years old or more. *Cornea.* 2013;32:602-607.
35. Kezirian GM, Stonecipher KG. Comparison of the Intralase femtosecond laser and mechanical keratotomy for laser in situ keratomileusis. *J Cataract Refract Surg.* 2004;30(4):804-811.
36. Binder PS. Flap dimensions created with the Intralase FS laser. *J Cataract Refract Surg.* 2004;30(4):26-32.
37. Lu Y, Chen X, Yang L, Xue C, Huang Z. Femtosecond laser-assisted deep anterior lamellar keratoplasty with big-bubble technique for keratoconus. *Indian J Ophthalmol.* 2016;64(9):639-642.
38. Chen G, Tzekov R, Li W, Jiang F, Mao S, Tong Y. Deep anterior lamellar keratoplasty versus penetrating keratoplasty: a meta-analysis of randomized controlled trials. *Cornea.* 2016;35:169-174
39. Sarnicola V, Toro P. Blunt cannula for descemetic deep anterior lamellar keratoplasty. *Cornea.* 2011;30(8):985-988.
40. Sogutlu Sari E, Kubaloglu A, Unal M, et al. Deep anterior lamellar keratoplasty versus penetrating keratoplasty for macular corneal dystrophy: a randomized trial. *Am J Ophthalmol.* 2013;156:267-274.
41. Spadea L, De Rosa V. Current techniques of lamellar keratoplasty for keratoconus. *Saudi Med J.* 2016;37(2):127-36.
42. Urrets-Zavalia A. Fixed dilated pupil, iris atrophy and secondary glaucoma: a distinct clinical entity following penetrating keratoplasty for keratoconus. *Am J Ophthalmol.* 1963;56:257-265.

43. Tan, DT, Dart JK, Holland EJ, Kinoshita S. Corneal transplantation. *Lancet.* 2012;379:1749-1761.
44. Arenas E, Esquenazi S, Anwar M, Terry M. Lamellar corneal transplantation. *Surv Ophthalmol.* 2012;57:510-529.
45. Keane MD, Coster M, Ziaei KW. Deep anterior lamellar keratoplasty versus penetrating keratoplasty for treating keratoconus. *Cochrane Database Syst.* 2014;(7):CD009700.
46. Reinhart WJ , Musch DC, Jacobs DS, Lee WB, Kaufman SC, Shtein RM. Deep anterior lamellar keratoplasty as an alternative to penetrating keratoplasty a report by the American Academy of Ophthalmology. *Ophthalmology.* 2011;118(1):209-218.
47. Shi JL, Feng YF, Yu JG, Wang QM. Meta analysis of deep lamellar keratoplasty and penetrating keratoplasty for keratoconus. *Chin J Exp Ophthalmol.* 2012;30(10):926-931.
48. Henein C, Nanavaty MA. Systematic review comparing penetrating keratoplasty and deep anterior lamellar keratoplasty for management of keratoconus. *Cont Lens Anterior Eye.* 2017;40(1):3-14.
49. Kim KH, Choi SH, Ahn K, Chung ES, Chung TY. Comparison of refractive changes after deep anterior lamellar keratoplasty and penetrating keratoplasty for keratoconus. *Jpn J Ophthalmol.* 2011;55:93-97.
50. Khattak A, Nakhli FR, Al-Arfaj KM, Cheema AA. Comparison of outcomes and complications of deep anterior lamellar keratoplasty and penetrating keratoplasty performed in a large group of patients with keratoconus. *Int Ophthalmol.* 2018;38(3):985-992.
51. Abdelkader A. Influence of different keratoplasty techniques on the biomechanical properties of the cornea. *Acta Ophthalmol.* 2013;91(7):e567-e572.
52. Shimazaki J. The evolution of lamellar keratoplasty. *Curr Opin Ophthalmol.* 2000;11:217-223.
53. Muraine M, Sanchez C, Watt L, Retout A, Brasseur G. Long-term results of penetrating keratoplasty. A 10-year-plus retrospective study. *Graefes Arch Clin Exp Ophthalmol.* 2003;241(7):571-576.
54. Brierly SC, Izquierdo L Jr, Mannis MJ. Penetrating keratoplasty for keratoconus. *Cornea.* 2000;19(3):329-32.
55. Fukuoka S, Honda N, Ono K, Mimura T, Usui T, Amano S. Extended long-term results of penetrating keratoplasty for keratoconus. *Cornea.* 2010;29(5):528-530.
56. Bilgihan K, Ozdek SC, Sari A, Hasanreisoglu B. Excimer laser-assisted anterior lamellar keratoplasty for keratoconus, corneal problems after laser in situ keratomileusis, and corneal stromal opacities. *J Cataract Refract Surg.* 2006;32(8):1264-1269.
57. Mosca L, Fasciani R, Tamburelli C, et al. Femtosecond laser-assisted lamellar keratoplasty: early results. *Cornea.* 2008;27(6):668-672.
58. Chan CC, Ritenour RJ, Kumar RL, Sansanayudh W, Rootman DS. Femtosecond laser-assisted mushroom configuration deep anterior lamellar keratoplasty. *Cornea.* 2010;29(3):290-295.
59. Lu Y, Yang L, Ge Y, Chen X, Huang Z. Femtosecond laser-assisted anterior lamellar keratoplasty for the treatment of stromal corneal pathology. *BMC Ophthalmol.* 2015;1(15):15.

Please see videos on the accompanying website at
www.healio.com/books/DALKvideos

3

Evaluation of the Patient and Decision Making in Anterior Lamellar Keratoplasty

Ashiyana Nariani, MD, MPH; Terry Kim, MD; Melissa B. Daluvoy, MD; and Alan N. Carlson, MD

Since the work done by Eduard Zirm in 1905 with the first successful human full-thickness penetrating keratoplasty (PK),[1] there have been several surgeons, including von Hippel,[2] Paufique and Charles,[3] McGhee, Kim, and Wilson,[4] and Anwar,[5] who have innovated lamellar corneal transplant surgery as a potential alternative to PK for a variety of indications (Table 3-1).[5-10]

Advantages

Deep anterior lamellar keratoplasty (DALK) has emerged in recent years as a preferred approach to conserve the host endothelium and to avoid rejection.[4] A report by the American Academy of Ophthalmology, in which 11 published studies comparing DALK with PK were analyzed, substantiated that DALK is superior to PK for preservation of endothelial cell density (ECD), avoiding risk of endothelial cell immune graft rejection and has additional theoretic safety advantages. There was no significant difference in best spectacle-corrected visual acuity, spherocylindrical refraction, nor postoperative astigmatism.[5-14]

Additional advantages of DALK over PK include enhanced structural integrity with less risk of rupture post-trauma,[15-20] faster recovery time with earlier visual improvement,[21] absence of endothelial graft rejection, increased intraocular stability during surgery,[22] reduced risk of choroidal hemorrhage and endophthalmitis, absence of need of donor graft with good endothelial count, better long-term graft survival,[23] no late failures, minimal steroid-related complications and easier follow-up.[5,24]

Jacob S, ed. *Mastering DALK: A Video Textbook on Deep Anterior Lamellar Keratoplasty* (pp 27-36).

Table 3-1

Indications for and Contraindications to Deep Anterior Lamellar Keratoplasty

Indications	Contraindications
• Ectasia: Keratoconus, keratoglobus, pellucid marginal degeneration,[25] post-refractive ectasia • Superficial corneal dystrophies: Epithelial (epithelial basement membrane dystrophy, Meesmann), Bowman's membrane (Reis-Bucklers', Thiel-Behnke), stroma (granular, lattice, macular) • Corneal degenerations and deposits: Salzmann's nodular degeneration, band keratopathy • Superficial corneal scars	• Break in Descemet's membrane (DM): Hydrops (the newly described Jacob modified technique of pre-Descemetic DALK [PD-DALK] may be performed as immediate primary management of acute hydrops to avoid scarring) • Corneal dystrophies involving endothelium: Fuchs', macular corneal dystrophy, congenital hereditary endothelial dystrophy, posterior polymorphous corneal dystrophy • Endothelial disease: Pseudophakic bullous keratopathy • Deep corneal scars involving DM and endothelium

Disadvantages

Despite the advantages of the DALK procedure, the technical challenges of and additional time required for the procedure prevent some surgeons from attempting it. Some argue that higher-order aberrations and light scatter caused by the surgical interface may be factors limiting post-DALK visual outcomes.[26]

In order to optimize resource expenditure, it is critical to understand the indications for and contraindications to performing DALK. For those patients where both DALK and PK are viable surgical options, DALK should be attempted as the benefits of attempting the DALK procedure outweigh the risks and is in the best interest of the patient.

Indications

DALK is the preferred corneal transplant procedure of choice, over PK, for the optical correction of axial corneal diseases with intact DM and healthy corneal

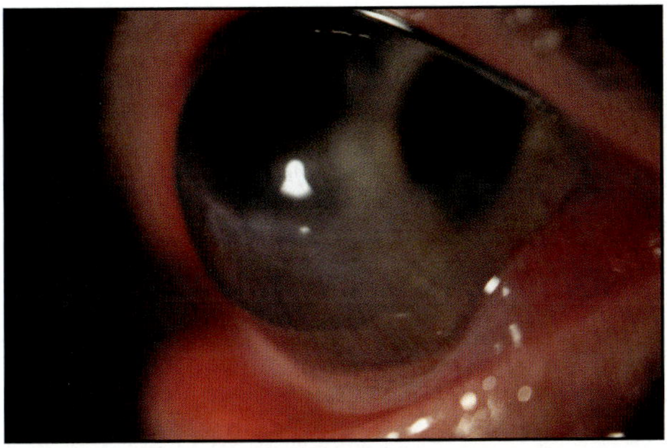

Figure 3-1. Keratoglobus. (Reprinted with permission from Melissa B. Daluvoy, MD, Duke University Eye Center, Durham, NC.)

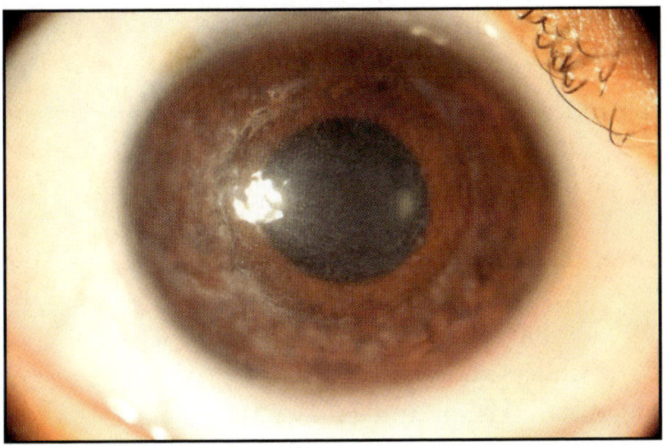

Figure 3-2. Lattice corneal dystrophy. (Reprinted with permission from Melissa B. Daluvoy, MD, Duke University Eye Center, Durham, NC.)

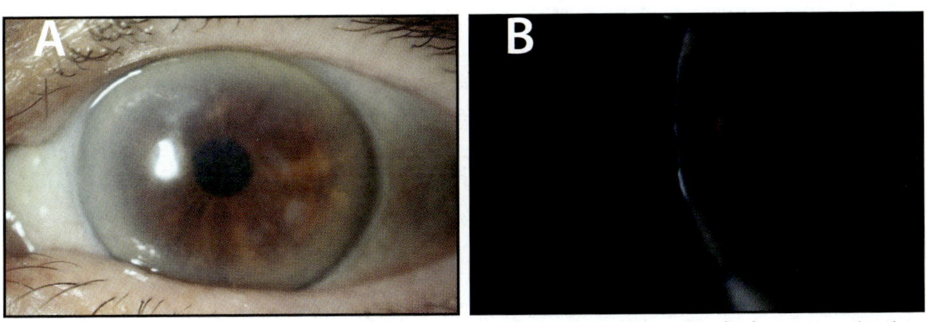

Figure 3-3. (A) Salzmann's nodular degeneration with corresponding (B) slit lamp examination. Reprinted with permission from Melissa B. Daluvoy, MD, Duke University Eye Center, Durham, NC.)

endothelium (see Table 3-1).[5-10] Indications can be classified into the following categories: ectasia (Figure 3-1), superficial corneal dystrophies (Figure 3-2), corneal degenerations (Figure 3-3) and deposits (Figure 3-4), and superficial corneal scars.[11]

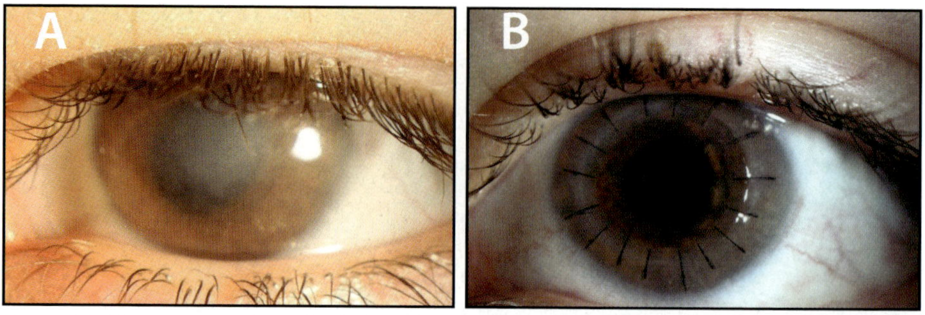

Figure 3.4. Cloudy cornea due to Hurler's syndrome (Mucopolysaccharidosis Type 1). (A) Preoperative and (B) postoperative after DALK procedure. (Reprinted with permission from Melissa B. Daluvoy, MD, Duke University Eye Center, Durham, NC.)

Special Considerations

Beyond the previously mentioned indications, there are special cases in patients with healthy endothelium where DALK is the definitive treatment of choice. Surgeons not performing DALK should refer to seasoned DALK surgeons the following case scenarios:

- Given the additional benefit of not having to use long-term steroids with the DALK procedure, it should be the procedure of choice particularly for patients who have normal endothelium but have any of the following factors at play:
  - Patients who are steroid responders and/or are phakic
  - Patients with poor compliance to therapy and follow-ups[6]
  - Patients at a higher risk of complications, such as positive pressure, iris prolapse, choroidal effusion/hemorrhage
- DALK has the theoretical advantage of less severity in dehisced suture wounds as compared to PK wounds; therefore, it may be preferred over PK in patients who are predisposed to ocular trauma (eg, personnel in the armed forces, those participating in contact sports).
- DALK has advantages of avoiding the intraocular, open-sky segment of the PK procedure, thereby avoiding complications. Patients residing in an area with harsh and severe climate, making them more prone to ocular surface disease due to environmental factors, would also benefit from undergoing a DALK when indicated as the risk of rejection in consequent vascularized corneas with pannus would be higher with a PK in place.
- Sutures may be removed earlier following DALK, allowing for potentially quicker refractive stability. This is important for younger patients at risk for amblyopia, as well as patients who are non-verbal or those with intellectual disabilities, such as patients with Down syndrome.
- Additional clinical scenarios where a DALK would be safer than a PK include keratoconus associated with inflammation (ie, vernal keratoconjunctivitis, monocular status, history of repeated graft rejections in the other eye).[6,7]

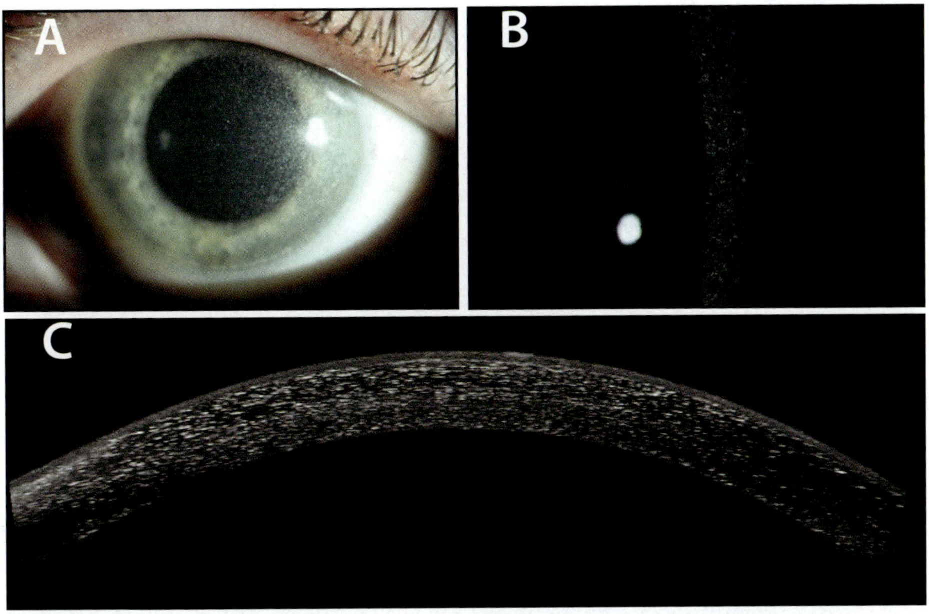

Figure 3-5. (A) Corneal cystinosis deposits, extending through all corneal layers on (B) slit lamp examination and (C) anterior segment optical coherence tomography (ASOCT). (Reprinted with permission from Melissa B. Daluvoy, MD, Duke University Eye Center, Durham, NC.)

Contraindications

The major contraindications to DALK are conditions where the DM or endothelium are diseased or unhealthy. These contraindications can be classified into the following categories (see Table 3-1):

- Breaks in DM—hydrops. It should be noted however that the Jacob modified technique of PD-DALK as a primary procedure for the treatment of acute hydrops is possible and has been reported to give excellent results in all cases[27,28] while avoiding scar formation, unlike conventional management techniques such as intracameral gas injection and compression sutures. This technique has been described in detail elsewhere in this book. DALK is also done routinely as a secondary procedure for post-hydrops scarring not involving the visual axis.
- Corneal dystrophies involving endothelium, endothelial disease, and deep corneal scars involving the DM and endothelium.
- Other examples include patients having keratoconus with coexisting Fuchs' endothelial dystrophy, cystinosis with progression to endothelial involvement (Figure 3-5), patients with corneal scarring, such as from herpes simplex virus, varicella zoster virus, microbial corneal ulcers involving the DM (Figure 3-6), and macular corneal dystrophy.[6,7]

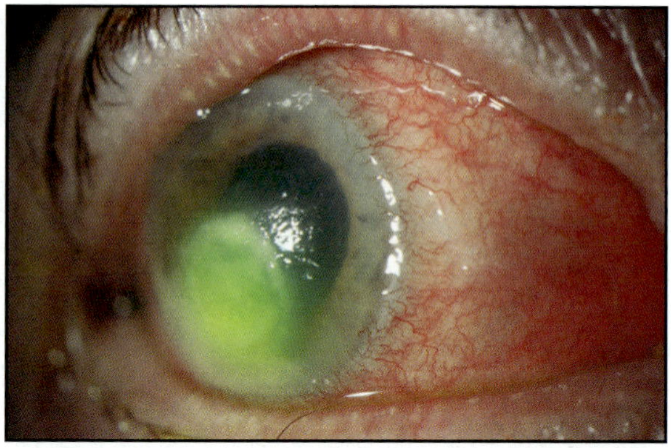

Figure 3-6. Corneal ulcer with anterior chamber hypopyon. (Reprinted with permission from Melissa B. Daluvoy, MD, Duke University Eye Center, Durham, NC.)

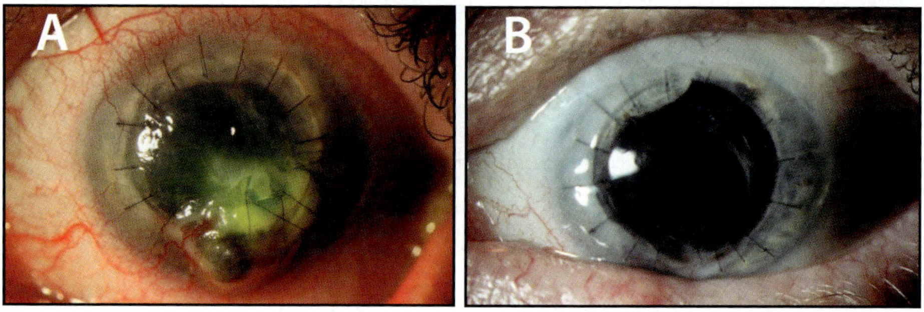

Figure 3-7. (A) Uveal prolapse through prior PK and (B) postoperative repeat PK. (Reprinted with permission from Melissa B. Daluvoy, MD, Duke University Eye Center, Durham, NC.)

- Patients with penetrating ocular trauma are generally not candidates for big bubble DALK (Figure 3-7), though this could be done as a PD-DALK if the scar does not involve the DM in the visual axis. Some eyes with deep stromal scarring may not have success with Descemet's-baring procedures due to the increased difficulty with deep stromal dissection.[24]

DALK may also be performed with variations in surgical technique in conditions such as keratoglobus, macular corneal dystrophy, descemetocele, and pellucid marginal degeneration.[11]

Preoperative Surgical Planning

Careful surgical planning and appropriate patient counseling lay the foundation for a successful outcome and a happy patient. A thorough history is important to understand the etiology of a corneal opacity (ie, herpetic scar vs hydrops with a break in DM), to gauge the chronicity of the condition and whether there are any special considerations that may affect the choice of intervention, as discussed previously. Assess systemic conditions (eg, diabetes mellitus, pregnancy, autoimmune conditions, HIV, and other immunocompromised states), ocular comorbidities (eg, herpes, dry eyes, blepharitis, eyelid malposition, glaucoma, cataract, retinopathy), prior ocular surgery, medications, and allergies. Check prior contact lens history and whether the patient will be able to tolerate contact lens wear postoperatively and be compliant with long-term topical steroids.

The work-up evaluation should include determining visual potential with a potential acuity meter, retinal acuity meter, or in uncooperative patients, with a visual evoked potential. A preoperative rigid gas permeable contact lens trial will further guide on whether or not the patient is likely to achieve an improvement in visual acuity postoperatively. If the view to the posterior segment is limited, perform a B-scan ultrasound to rule out posterior segment pathology.

The surgeon must be cognizant of the health of the endothelium, the corneal layers through which the opacity extends, whether the opacity is central or peripheral, the dimensions of the opacity and whether or not the DM is intact. For these assessments, a thorough slit lamp examination is critical. Specular microscopy is a useful adjunct for ECD and health. ASOCT imaging will provide insight into the depth, location, and dimensions of the corneal opacity as well as pachymetry (see Figure 3-5). Corneal topography and pachymetry can provide data on the level and location of corneal steepening and thinning, to help predict inadequate vacuum suction during trephination, the possibility of not achieving the desired dissection and the possibility of making a penetrating cut with the trephine.[29]

The surgical technique used will be determined by which corneal layers will need to be removed to optimize vision and interface clarity. For corneal pathology or opacities involving the superficial and mid-stromal layers, proceed with a superficial anterior lamellar keratoplasty.[30,31] If DM is compromised by past hydrops, perforation or other forms of scarring, deep dissection techniques, such as Anwar's big bubble technique, are more likely to result in Descemet's rupture and conversion to PK. These patients may benefit from a PD-DALK procedure with manual dissection.[32] Hydrops may also be managed in the acute stage with the Jacob modified technique of PD-DALK to prevent stromal scarring as well as obtain topographic, biomechanical, structural, and visual improvement and decreased contact lens dependence while avoiding 2 surgeries[27,28] as well as avoiding the risk of scarring over the visual axis necessitating a PK.

If the pathology has posterior stromal involvement as well, consider a DALK, involving removal of the posterior stroma. Finally, for full-thickness pathology involving DM over the visual axis or with endothelial compromise, proceed with a full-thickness PK. A full-thickness scar not over the visual axis with healthy endothelium may be tackled with a PD-DALK. The decision making between these procedures is important as both DALK and PK eyes achieve similar visual results, with quicker return of vision and often one or two lines of better visual acuity as compared to PD-DALK.[33,34] This textbook will provide in-depth knowledge on each of these procedures in later chapters.

Patient Counseling

Based on preoperative planning, evaluation, and work-up, the surgeon and surgical team can proceed with appropriate patient counseling and informed consent. Patients planned for a DALK, must be informed on the technical challenges of the procedure and the possibility of a DM perforation and conversion to a PK. The risks of infection, need for additional procedures, and need for repeating the procedure in the future exist, similar to patients undergoing a PK, and need to be discussed. In both DALK and PK patients, vision is limited by unpredictable refractive error and irregular astigmatism. Extensive postoperative follow-up is required with staged removal of sutures. Patients should understand the need for glasses or contact lenses following surgery, and possibly even refractive surgery for high levels of spherocylindrical errors. Duration of visual rehabilitation as well as the long-term use of topical steroids should be emphasized to both the patient and family prior to surgery. Additionally, outcomes of DALK are often related to the underlying diagnosis and indication for surgery, including visual, tectonic, and ocular surface disease as well as the often coexistent allergic eye disease. Goals of care and visual prognosis should also be discussed and ocular comorbidities should be treated. Nevertheless, the advantages of the DALK procedure, including the safety of a relatively closed system and the reduced long-term risk of visual loss from rejection, are key features of electing to proceed with DALK as compared to a PK, and these benefits should indeed be highlighted.[29]

Donor Tissue Selection

The DALK donor tissue does not require healthy endothelium and can be obtained from the eye bank accordingly. However, PK tissue with healthy endothelium should be readily available due to the potential need to convert to PK should a significant DM rupture occur. One donor graft can potentially be split for DM endothelial keratoplasty and DALK, so planning one's case schedule can be made accordingly to make donor tissue usage efficient.[35]

Anesthesia Considerations

Lamellar keratoplasty can, and often is, performed under local anesthetic; however, monitoring by an anesthesiologist or designate is advised. General anesthesia is useful for a surgeon learning the technique; however, as air may be used in the anterior chamber, the anesthetist must be informed that no nitrous oxide should be used, as this will result in expansion of the air bubble within the eye. The latter may have unexpected and serious consequences, including high pressure and loss of vision.[29]

Conclusion

Patient selection is critical to avoid wastage of operating room resources, time, and money. As visual acuity does not differ between PK and DALK, the benefits of DALK, namely lack of endothelial immune reaction and increased ocular stability, outweigh the risk of additional complications and DALK should, therefore, be performed whenever possible and indicated.[36]

References

1. Firm EK. [A successful total keratoplasty]. *Refract Corneal Sure.* 1989;5:258-261.
2. von Hippel A. Eine neue Methode der Hornhauttransplantation. *Graefes Arch Ophthalmol.* 1888;34:108-130.
3. Paufique L, Charleux J. Lamellar keratoplasty. In: Casey T, ed. *Corneal Grafting.* London, United Kingdom: Butterworth; 1972:121-176.
4. McGhee CN, Kim BZ, Wilson PJ. Contemporary treatment paradigms in keratoconus. *Cornea.* 2015; 34(suppl 10):S16-S23.
5. Anwar M. Technique in lamellar keratoplasty. *Trans Ophthalmol Soc UK.* 1947;94:163-171.
6. Reinhart WJ, Busch DC, Jacobs DS, Lee B, Kaufman SC, Stein RM. Deep anterior lamellar keratoplasty as an alternative to penetrating keratoplasty. *Ophthalmology.* 2011;118:209-218.
7. Keane M, Coster D, Ziaei M, Williams K. Deep anterior lamellar keratoplasty versus penetrating keratoplasty for treating keratoconus. *Cochrane Database Syst Rev.* 2014;(7):CD009700.
8. Henein C, Nanavaty MA. Systematic review comparing penetrating keratoplasty and deep anterior lamellar keratoplasty for management of keratoconus. *Cont Lens Anterior Eye.* 2017;40(1):3-14.
9. Han DCY, Mehta JS, Por YM, et al. Comparison of outcomes of lamellar keratoplasty and penetrating keratoplasty in keratconus. *Am J Ophthalmol.* 2009;148:744-51.
10. Fontana L, Parente G, Sincich A, et al. Influence of graft-host interface on the quality of vision after deep anterior lamellar keratoplasty in patients with keratoconus. *Am J Ophthalmol.* 2007;143:117-24.
11. Anwar, M. Indications for anterior lamellar keratoplasty In: Krachmer JH, Mannis MJ, Holland EJ, eds. *Cornea: Surgery of the Cornea and Conjunctiva. Volume 2.* 3rd ed. Amsterdam, Netherlands: Elsevier; 2010.
12. Anwar M. Planned near Descemet's membrane dissection using air and fluid. In: John T, ed. *Surgical Techniques in Anterior and Posterior Lamellar Corneal Surgery.* New Delhi, India: Jaypee Brothers; 2006:126-133.
13. Mahmood MA, Wagoner MD. Penetrating keratoplasty in eyes with keratoconus and vernal keratoconjunctivitis. *Cornea.* 2000;19:468-470.
14. Anwar M. Big-bubble technique. In: Fontana L, Tassinari G, eds. *Atlas of Lamellar Keratoplasty.* Moasca, Italy: Fabiano Editore; 2007:125-136.
15. Zarei-Ghanavati S, Zarei-Ghanavati M, Sheibani S. Traumatic wound dehiscence after deep anterior lamellar keratoplasty protective role of intact Descemet's membrane after big-bubble technique. *Cornea.* 2010;29(2):220-221.
16. Prasher P, Muftuoglu O, Mootha VV. Traumatic graft dehiscence after anterior lamellar keratoplasty. *Cornea.* 2009;28(2):240-242.
17. Lee WB, Mathys KC. Traumatic wound dehiscence after deep anterior lamellar keratoplasty. *J Cataract Refract Surg.* 2009; 35(6):1129-1131.
18. Kawashima M, Kawakita T, Shimmura S, Tsubota K, Shimazaki J. Characteristics of traumatic globe rupture after keratoplasty. *Ophthalmology.* 2009;116(1):2072-2076.
19. Fiorentzis M, Baurle S, Viestenz A, Seitz B, Viestenz A. Traumatic globe rupture after deep anterior lamellar keratoplasty—a novel management technique. *Clin Anat.* 2018;31(1):56-59.

20. Meyer JJ, McGhee CN. Incidence, severity and outcomes of traumatic wound dehiscence following penetrating keratoplasty and deep anterior lamellar keratoplasty. *Br J Ophthalmol.* 2016;100(1):1412-1415.
21. Yuksel B, Kandemir B, Uzunel UD, Celik O, Ceylan S, Kusbeci T. Comparison of visual and topographic outcomes of deep-anterior lamellar keratoplasty and penetrating keratoplasty in keratoconus. *Int J Ophthalmol.* 2017;10(3):385-390.
22. Cursiefen C, Schaub F, Bachmann B. Update: deep anterior lamellar keratoplasty (DALK) for keratoconus. When, how and why. *Ophthalmologe.* 2016;113(3):204-212.
23. Borderie VM, Boelle PY, Touzeau O, Allouch C, Boutboul S, Laroche L. Predicted long-term outcome of corneal transplantation. *Ophthalmology.* 2009;116(12):2354-2360.
24. Vickers L, Kim T. Deep anterior lamellar keratoplasty. In: Agarwal A, John T, ed. *Mastering Corneal Surgery: Recent Advances and Current Techniques.* Thorofare, NJ: SLACK Incorporated; 2015:41-52.
25. Moshirfar M, Edmonds JN, Behunin NL, Christiansen SM. Current options in the management of pellucid marginal degeneration. *J Refract Surg.* 2014;30(7):474-485.
26. Feizi S, Javadi MA, Mohammad-Rabei H. Analysis of factors influencing quality of vision after big-bubble deep anterior lamellar keratoplasty in keratoconus. *Am J Ophthalmol.* 2016;162:66-73.
27. Jacob S, Narasimhan S, Agarwal A, Sambath J, Umamaheshwari G, Saijimol AI. Primary modified predescemetic deep anterior lamellar keratoplasty in acute corneal hydrops. *Cornea.* 2018;37(10):1328-1333.
28. Jacob S. Primary predescemetic DALK for acute hydrops Soosan Jacob with audio [video]. YouTube. https://www.youtube.com/watch?v=5ZeAXOmVDJw. Published June 14, 2018. Accessed September 27, 2018.
29. Daya SM, Hamada S. Deep anterior lamellar keratoplasty. In: Brightbill FS, McDonnell PJ, McGee CNJ, Farjo AA, Serdarevic ON, eds. *Corneal Surgery: Theory, Technique and Tissue.* 4th ed. Amsterdam, Netherlands: Elsevier: 2009:353-364.
30. Patel AK, Scorcia V, Kadyan A, Lapenna L, Ponzin D, Busin M. Microkeratome-assisted superficial anterior lamellar keratoplasty for anterior stromal corneal opacities after penetrating keratoplasty. *Cornea.* 2012;31(1):101-105.
31. Fogla R, Knyazer B. Microkeratome-assisted two-stage technique of superficial anterior lamellar keratoplasty for Reis-Bücklers corneal dystrophy. *Cornea.* 2014;33(10):1118-1122.
32. Chew ACY, Mehta JS, Tan DTH. Deep lamellar keratoplasty after resolution of hydrops in keratoconus. *Cornea.* 2011;30(4);454-459.
33. Adrjomand N, Has S, McAlister JC, et al. Quality of vision and graft thickness in deep anterior lamellar and penetrating corneal allografts. *Am J Ophthalmol.* 2007; 143:228-235.
34. Sarnicola V, Toro P, Gentile D, Hannush SB. Descemetic DALK and predescemetic DALK: outcomes in 236 cases of keratoconus. *Cornea.* 2010;29(1):53-59.
35. Heindl LM, Riss S, Bachmann BO, et al. Split cornea transplantation for 2 recipients: a new strategy to reduce corneal tissue cost and shortage. *Ophthalmology.* 2011;118:294-301.
36. Cursiefen C, Siebelmann S, Bachmann B. Complications of deep anterior lamellar keratoplasty. Avoid, recognize and treat. *Ophthalmologe.* 2015;112(12):961-968.

Please see videos on the accompanying website at
www.healio.com/books/DALKvideos

4

Superficial Anterior Lamellar Keratoplasty

Mukesh Patil, MBBS, MD, FICO, FAICO;
Noopur Gupta, MBBS, MS, DNB, PhD; Murugesan Vanathi, MBBS, MD; and
Radhika Tandon, MBBS, MD, DNB, MNAMS, FRCS(Ed), FRCOphth, MNASI

Keratoplasty is a procedure to restore vision in patients who have lost the ability to focus light because of a loss of corneal transparency. Full-thickness penetrating keratoplasty (PK) has been the surgical modality of choice for various corneal pathologies over the past few decades[1,2]; however, it can be complicated by suture related complications, endothelial rejection with a subsequent possibility of graft failure, and use of long-term topical steroids.

More recently, lamellar keratoplasty has become the procedure of choice in which only affected corneal layers are selectively replaced by healthy lamellar donor tissue. In cases of anterior stromal opacities, anterior lamellar keratoplasty (ALK) targets the replacement of only the anterior stromal tissue preserving the endothelium and thereby obviating the risk of endothelial rejection. Suture-related factors account for 14% to 60% of graft infections, compromising graft survival after the keratoplasty.[3,4] These complications have been avoided with the use of human fibrin glue in what have been described as *sutureless anterior lamellar keratoplasty.*[5]

Superficial anterior lamellar keratoplasty (SALK), aided by the use of human fibrin glue, can be used in cases of anterior stromal opacities involving less than one-third of the anterior corneal stroma. The main advantages of ALK include decreased incidence of graft rejection, and reduced intraoperative complications associated with the full-thickness open-sky procedures.[6] Lately, improvement in instrumentation, surgical techniques, and automation have enhanced the surgical efficiency and visual and anatomical outcomes following ALK surgery. Newer studies have confirmed that the visual outcomes of ALK are comparable to the results of PK.[7]

Jacob S, ed. *Mastering DALK: A Video Textbook on Deep Anterior Lamellar Keratoplasty* (pp 37-49).

Table 4-1

Indications for and Contraindications to Superficial Anterior Lamellar Keratoplasty

Indications	Contraindications
• Post-keratitis scars • Post-traumatic scars • Salzmann nodular degeneration • Epithelial-stromal TGFBI dystrophies • Stromal dystrophies • Trachomatous keratopathy • Post–chemical injury scars • Severe scarring after photorefractive keratectomy (PRK) • Recurrent epithelial ingrowth after LASIK	• Deep scars involving more than one-third of the anterior corneal stroma • Corneal endothelial disorders • Uncontrolled glaucoma • Active uveitis • Ocular surface disorders • Eyes with small palpebral aperture • Deep-set eyes • Systemic conditions like uncontrolled diabetes, collagen vascular disease, and immunocompromising conditions

Clinical Applications

The indications of SALK include the pathologies limited to anterior one-third of the corneal stroma (Table 4-1), such as in:

- *Post keratitis scars* (Figure 4-1): Keratitis could heal with either a nebular, macular, or leucomatous opacity. This technique could be very useful for such scars that are limited to the anterior one-third of the stromal depth.
- *Post-traumatic scars*: Trauma could also result in scars or opacities limited to the anterior layers of the cornea. The aforementioned techniques in such cases could minimize the risk of suture-related complications and provide a quick visual rehabilitation in such cases.
- *Salzmann nodular degeneration*: The degenerative changes are limited to the superficial layers of the cornea and a SALK comes handy in these cases to restore the vision.
- *Epithelial-stromal TGFBI dystrophies* (Figure 4-2): The pathology in these cases remains limited to the epithelium or the anterior stroma in depth. The opacities are quite superficial, rendering them easily amenable to SALK.

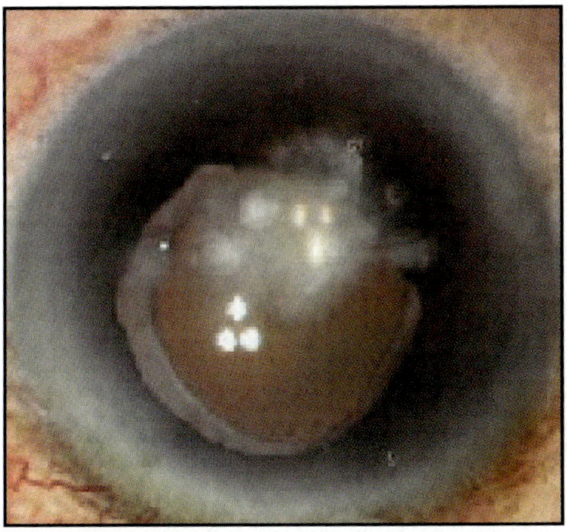

Figure 4-1. Post-keratitis scar.

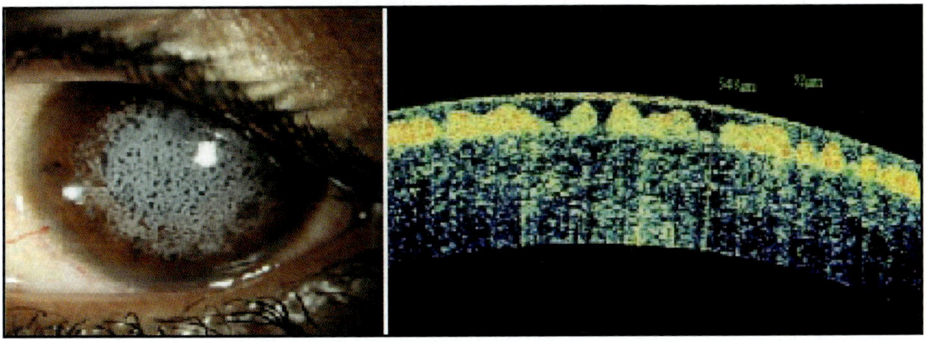

Figure 4-2. Epithelial-stromal TGFBI dystrophy.

- *Stromal dystrophies* (Figure 4-3): Stromal corneal dystrophies present with a varied involvement of the stromal depth. Hence, in cases where the opacities are limited to the anterior one-third of the cornea, this procedure could indeed be useful.
- *Trachomatous keratopathy*: Trachoma results in opacification of the superficial layers of the cornea resulting in loss of transparency of the cornea and poor quality of vision. SALK in such cases provides an enhanced quality of vision and faster recovery.
- *Post-chemical injury scars*: Chemical injuries resulting in superficial opacities form another indication for SALK.
- *Severe scarring after PRK*: An untoward complication of a refractive procedure such as PRK might result in superficial scarring and poorer postoperative visual outcomes. SALK in these cases provides a means of rescue to restore vision.
- *Recurrent epithelial ingrowth after laser in situ keratomileusis*[8,9]: Epithelial ingrowth with flap necrosis following LASIK procedure could, in rare and severe cases, require SALK following flap amputation.

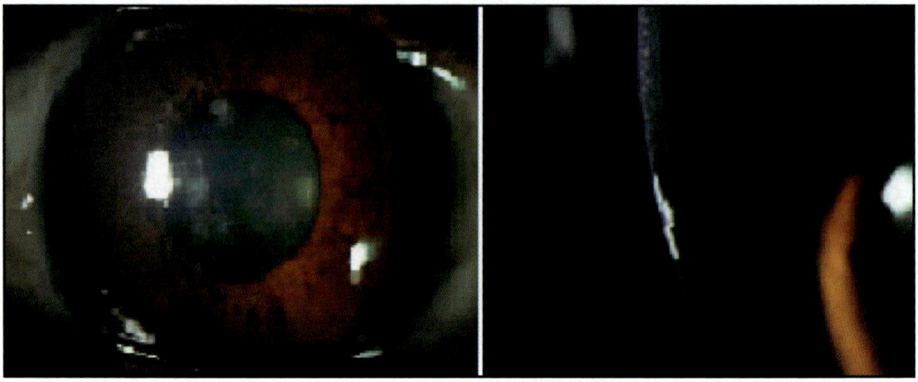

Figure 4-3. Stromal dystrophy.

Contraindications

The contraindications to SALK include the following:

- *Deep scars involving more than one-third of anterior corneal stroma*: Deeper scars are not amenable for dissection by superficial keratoplasty and may instead require either a deep lamellar or a full-thickness PK.
- *Corneal endothelial disorders*: As has been previously mentioned, a healthy endothelium is a prerequisite for any superficial keratoplasty procedure. In cases with a compromised endothelium, it is advisable to proceed with full-thickness PK.
- *Uncontrolled glaucoma*: Raised intraocular pressure (IOP) interferes with healing of the graft and can result in the primary failure of the graft.
- *Active uveitis*: Uveitis causes inflammation and can result in a failed graft.
- *Ocular surface disorders*: Dry eye disease and lid abnormalities, such as entropion, ectropion, and trichiasis, can result in failure of the graft by interfering with the healing process or causing recurrent breakdown of the tear film. Thus, the presence of any ocular surface abnormality is a relative contraindication for performing SALK until it is treated first.
- *Eyes with small palpebral aperture, deep-set eyes*: Eyes with small palpebral aperture and deep-set eyes pose difficulty in fitting of the microkeratome head over the host bed and thereby cause problems in preparation of the host bed.
- *Systemic conditions like uncontrolled diabetes, collagen vascular disease, and immunocompromising conditions*: These conditions can impair healing and uptake of the graft and hence systemic optimization is mandatory before any surgical procedure is planned in such cases.

Essentials of Surgical Technique

Preoperative Evaluation

It is indeed important to do a thorough preoperative evaluation before planning a patient for SALK. This includes a holistic elicitation of history as well as clinical examination. The history is important to know the exact nature and, if applicable, inheritance pattern of the pathology. The important aspects include any use of ocular or systemic medications, previous ocular surgery, occupation, and visual demands. It is also important to explain realistically the visual and anatomical outcomes and associated complications.

The systemic history and examination are important to rule out the presence of any collagen vascular diseases, diabetes mellitus, or any other immunocompromising conditions that might pose a difficulty for the survival of the graft.

The preoperative ocular examination includes the following:

- *Visual acuity*: Both the uncorrected and best-corrected visual acuity are to be noted. This could be done with the Snellen's, ETDRS (Early Treatment Diabetic Retinopathy Study), or logMAR visual acuity charts. Refraction and contact lens trial should be done wherever possible.
- *External eye examination*: Ocular surface and ocular adnexa should be thoroughly examined to look for the presence of any dry eye disease, entropion, ectropion, lagophthalmos, and trichiatic eye lashes. It is pertinent to rule out these pathologies as these could lead to delayed epithelialization and in turn decreased survival of the graft.
- *Slit lamp biomcroscopy*: Slit lamp examination includes the assessment of the tear film, the extent and depth of opacity, any other previous surgical scars, iris and lens status, and also the status of endothelium, as unhealthy endothelium precludes the possibility of ALK and in such cases a full-thickness PK should instead be planned.
- *Assessment for dry eye*: Tear film assessment is very important as healthy ocular surface is the key to the healing and survival of the graft. Tear film examination includes the tear film breakup time and the Schirmer's test.
- *IOP*: IOP should be measured preoperatively, and all measures should be taken to reduce the high IOP so as to allow timely epithelialization and healing of the graft.
- *Visual potential*: Preoperative assessment of the visual potential is recommended to aid in prognostication as the opacities may sometimes be long standing since early childhood, with the possibilities of preexisting amblyopia. The chances of postoperative visual gain in such cases are bleak. This includes a thorough fundus examination to rule out any comorbid retinal pathology. Other tests that could be done to assess visual potential are laser interferometry or potential acuity meter.

Special Investigations

Anterior Segment Optical Coherence Tomography

Anterior segment optical coherence tomography (ASOCT) helps to clearly find out the depth of opacity and is the most important tool in planning the surgery.

Pachymetry

The corneal thickness could be measured with either the optical or ultrasonic pachymetric methods. This measurement helps us to avoid inadvertent surgery and complications in cases of thinner corneas.

Specular Microscopy

Specular microscopy should be done to find out the status of host endothelium, as it is the prerequisite for performing ALK.

Confocal Scan

Confocal scan is an alternate tool that can help to assess the host endothelial status and to ascertain the depth of involvement.

Topography

The topographic analysis of the cornea is important to rule out any concurrent ectatic corneal disorder.

Surgical Technique

SALK can be done under local or general anesthesia depending on patient's age and cooperation. Various techniques of SALK are as follows:

- Microkeratome-assisted SALK
- Hemiautomated SALK
- Femtosecond laser–assisted SALK

Preparation of Host Bed

The host lamellar bed can either be prepared with microkeratome and the suction ring, superficial manual dissection, or the femtosecond-assisted dissection as has been mentioned previously. The advancement of the microkeratome over the suction ring can either be fully automated (ALK System; Figure 4-4) or be manually assisted (Gebauer Medizintechnik GmbH; Figure 4-5). The microkeratomes are available with different heads in which various ranges of blades can be fitted depending upon the desired depth of the cut. The aim of this maneuver is to cut a superficial corneal lamella with the same diameter and thickness as the donor tissue.

Dissection of superficial diseased host tissue can be done manually with the help of diamond knife and crescent blade (Figure 4-6). The host bed is then washed with

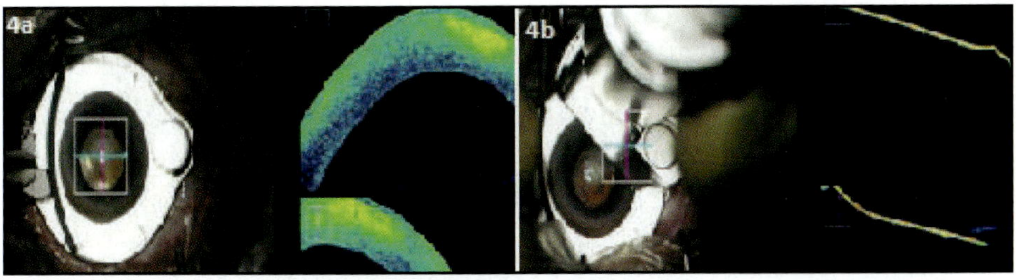

Figure 4-4. (A, B) Preparation of host bed with fully automated microkeratome (ALK System).

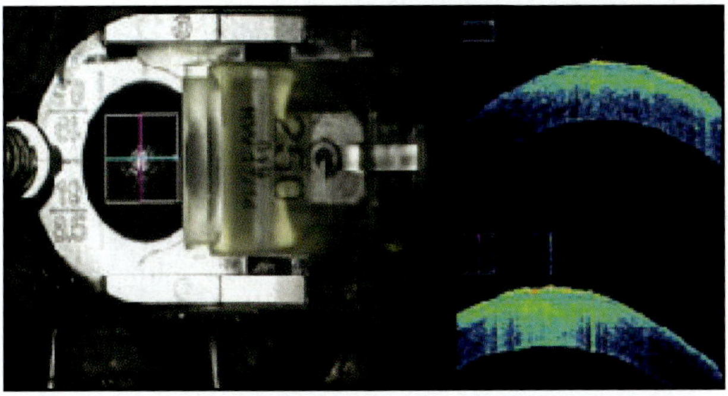

Figure 4-5. Preparation of host bed with manually advanced microkeratome (Gebauer Medizintechnik GmbH).

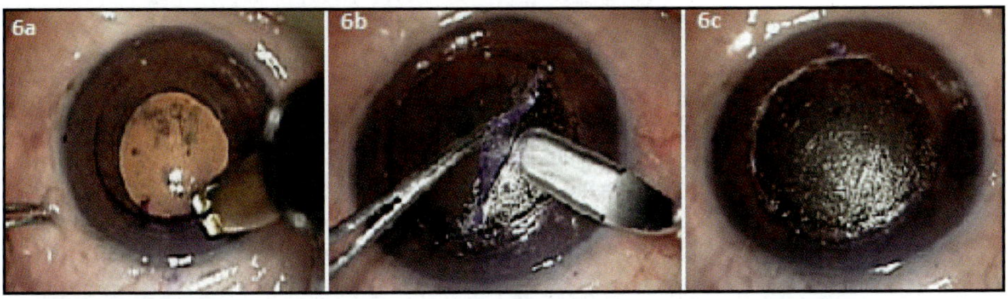

Figure 4-6. (A-C) Superficial dissection of stroma with diamond knife and crescent blade.

balanced salt solution (BSS) to remove any overlying debris. Never discard the dissected lamellar host tissue and keep it safely under aseptic conditions until surgery is over.

Preparation of Donor Lenticule

The ideal donor tissue is one with no or minimal arcus and an adequate rim of at least 2 to 3 mm for ease of mounting over the artificial anterior chamber (AAC). However, even a non–optical grade tissue can suffice, and an optical grade backup is not absolutely essential.

The donor corneal button can be prepared with the help of any of the readily available microkeratomes. The movement of microkeratome head is motor driven, which

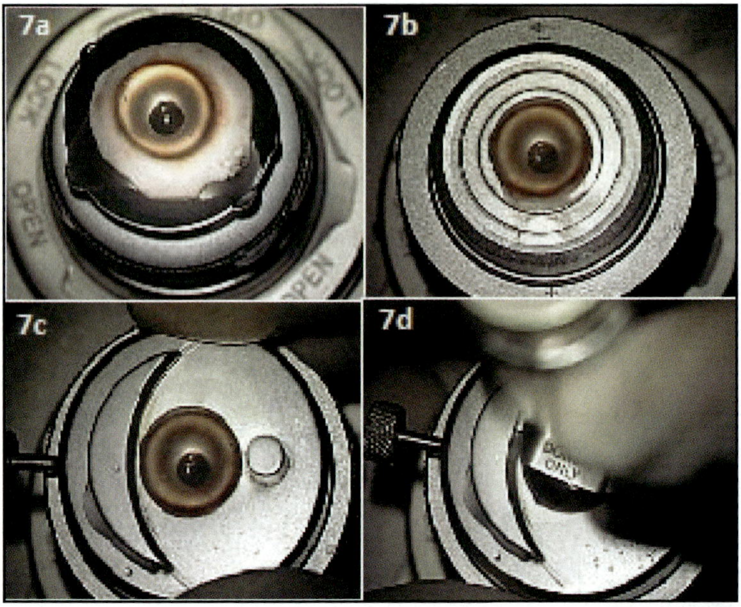

Figure 4-7. (A-D) Preparation of donor lenticule with manually advanced microkeratome (ALK System).

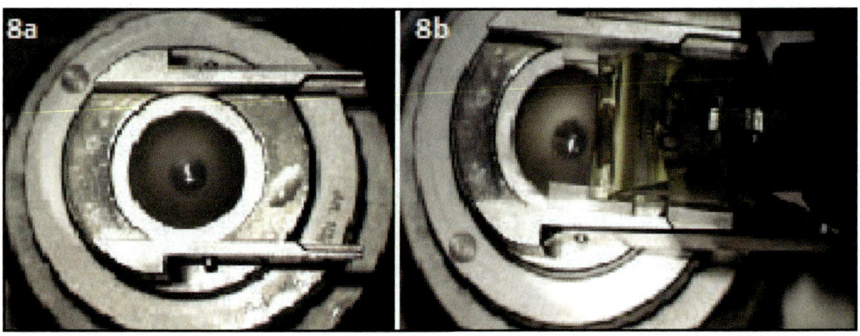

Figure 4-8. (A, B) Preparation of donor lenticule with fully-automated microkeratome (Gebauer Medizintechnik GmbH).

could either be manually assisted (ALK System; Figure 4-7) or totally automated (Gebauer Medizintechnik GmbH; Figure 4-8).

General principles of the microkeratome are universal among different models or manufacturers. Various prototypes differ to a lesser or greater extent in terms of certain specific aspects, such as the rotatory vs translational movements, speed of movement, extent of precision achievable in terms of various head sizes and blade parameters, source of power, console display, and foot switch design. For convenience, one prototype is described that is automated motor driven microkeratome. (Gebauer Medizintechnik GmbH). It has the following parts (Figure 4-9):

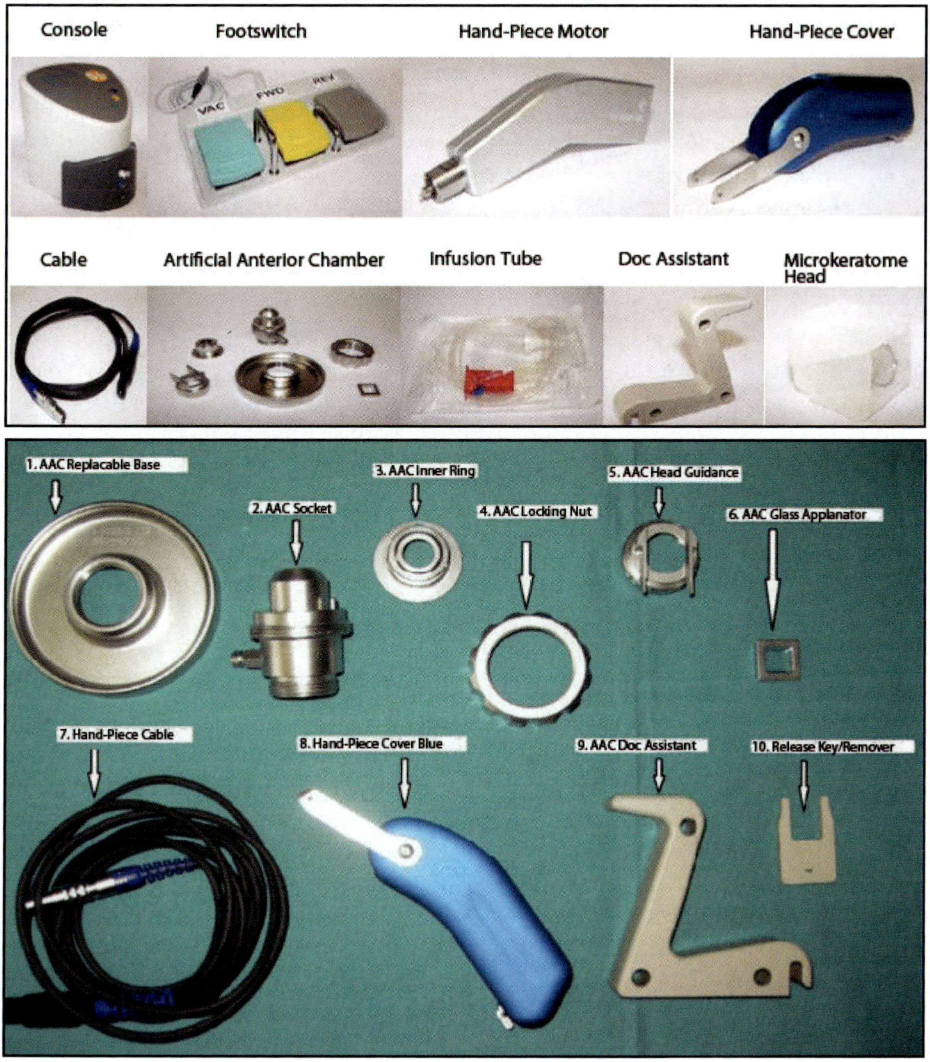

Figure 4-9. Parts of the automated motor driven microkeratome (Gebauer Medizintechnik GmbH).

- Console
- Footswitch
- Hand-piece motor
- Hand-piece cover
- Cable
- AAC
- Infusion tube
- Doc assistant
- Microkeratome head

The power cord is first connected to the back of Gebauer SLc console and is switched on and the footswitch is then connected to the front of Gebauer SLc console. Hand-piece motor is assembled to the hand-piece cover and the cable is connected to the hand-piece and to the front of console. Vacuum connection is locked with the dummy plug, and the BSS infusion bottle and tubing are attached to the infusion stand. This infusion tubing is connected to the AAC socket and the infusion is run until flow appears from the top of AAC socket. It is important to measure the BSS level in the infusion tube cylinder to the platform where the AAC is located and it is to be ensured that the right height is adjusted from the BSS level in cylinder, approximately 95 cm high to the AAC platform.

The donor tissue is placed on the AAC socket ensuring that there are no air bubbles present beneath the tissue while placing it, and the BSS infusion is closed. Now, place the AAC inner ring over the AAC socket with the pin in to hole configuration and secure this ring by rotating it clockwise until tight, and the infusion is now opened. The corneal thickness should be measured at this point using either hand-held pachymeter or intraoperative OCT. The microkeratome head is then chosen based upon the desired depth of cut and is connected to the hand-piece. The AAC head guidance is aligned with the thread of the AAC inner ring and is rotated clockwise (1/4 to 1/2 rotation only). The glass applanator is glided onto the AAC head guidance and the guidance is rotated clockwise until desired applanation is achieved (9.0/10.0 mm) and the hand-piece is loaded onto AAC.

The infusion tubing is locked and closed, and the vacuum is activated by pressing the VAC pedal once. An audible beep is heard and at this point, the cut is performed by pressing the FWD pedal constantly until another audible beep is heard. The REV pedal is then pressed constantly to return to start position and is terminated at the sound of audible beep. The vacuum is switched off and hand-piece is removed from the AAC with the aid of the release key. The superficial lamellar donor corneal button should be carefully and gently removed from the microkeratome head. The AAC head guidance is removed by rotating in a counterclockwise manner. The AAC lock nut is removed by rotating counterclockwise and infusion is switched on while gently lifting up the AAC inner ring. The donor corneal tissue can now be removed from inside the inner ring.

Donor Recipient Apposition

After thoroughly washing and drying the host bed to remove any debris, the fibrin glue (Tisseel kit VH; Baxter AG) can either be placed evenly on host stromal bed (Figure 4-10A) or it can be applied along the edges of the host tissue sparing the stromal bed. Then, the donor lenticule is placed over the host bed and is allowed to adhere. Bandage contact lens can be applied at the end of surgery (Figure 4-10B).

Postoperative Treatment and Follow Up

A postoperative antibiotic-steroid regimen is prescribed along with lubricant drops for faster epithelization and no or minimal interface haze. Steroids are

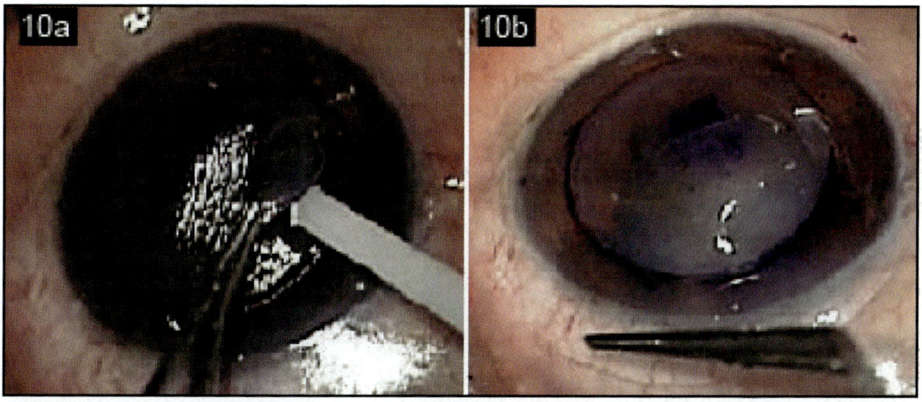

Figure 4-10. (A) Fibrin glue–assisted donor recipient apposition. Glue is applied in the interface. (B) Donor lenticule is placed over host bed and is allowed to adhere. Bandage contact lens can be applied at the end of surgery.

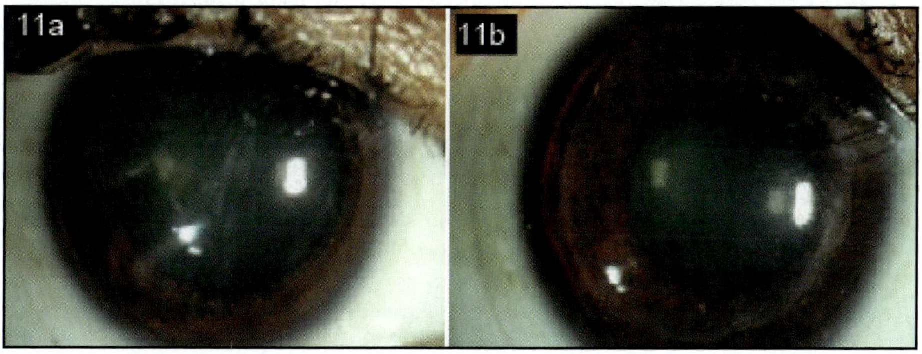

Figure 4-11. (A) A 32-year-old female patient developed nebulo-macular corneal opacity involving visual axis following road traffic accident. (B) ASOCT revealed involvement up to 160 μm and patient successfully underwent SALK procedure with good postoperative vision gain.

subsequently tapered. Bandage contact lens can be removed after complete epithelization is achieved, which usually takes 1 to 2 weeks (Figures 4-11 and 4-12).

Complications

Complications associated with this procedure can either be intraoperative or postoperative.

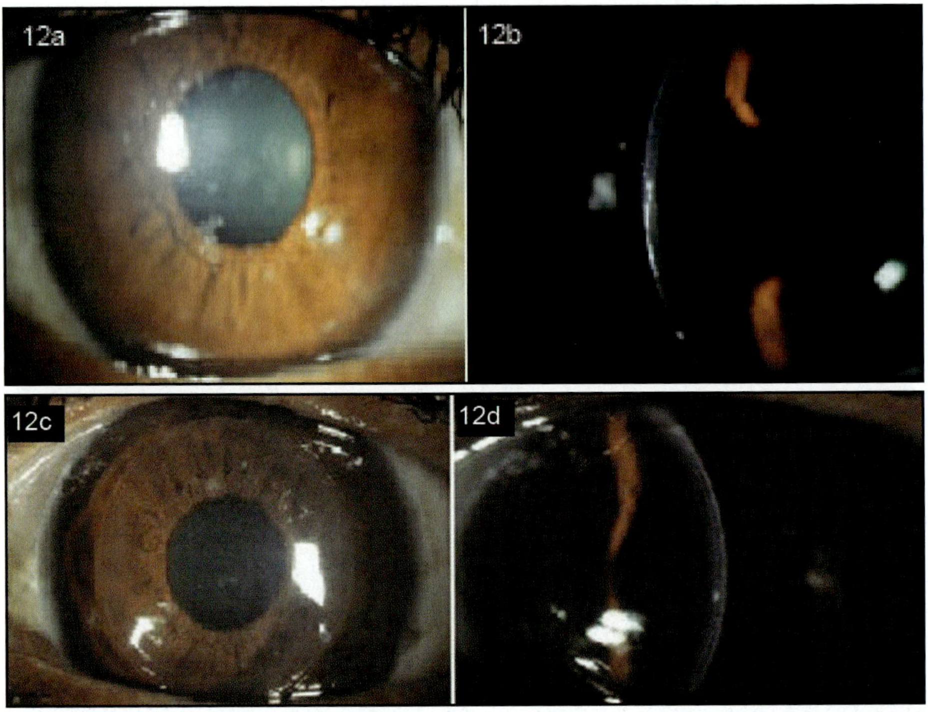

Figure 4-12. (A, B) A 38-year-old female patient with granular corneal dystrophy presented with gradual diminution of vision. Examination finding showed involvement of superficial stroma. (C, D) SALK was performed with better visual outcome and decreased symptoms.

Intraoperative Complications

These are mainly microkeratome-related complications. Such complications mainly occur during host bed preparation and include loss of suction or difficulty in movement of microkeratome, especially in deep set eyes. This can result in formation of partial flap due to incomplete pass.

Other important complications related to use of microkeratome are the mismatch between the size of host and donor tissues. This mainly occurs as the flap diameters are not predicable and can be managed with the adjunctive use of anchoring sutures or tucking of the graft in the host rim or by adequately sized trephination of the graft. These problems are, however, minimized with the advent of femtosecond laser–assisted flaps. This is because the size and thickness of the femtosecond flaps are precise and hence the apposition problems are minimal.[10] Rarely, perforation of host tissue can occur in cases of localized thinning or in corneal ectatic disorders.

Postoperative Complications

The most important complications include the following[5,11]:

- Graft dislocation
- Graft infection
- Epithelial ingrowth
- Vascularization
- Recurrence of primary pathology
- Graft rejection
- Regular and irregular astigmatism
- Interface haze
- Residual corneal opacity
- Glare, halos, and decreased contrast sensitivity
- Steroid-induced glaucoma

The SALK procedure has limited indications, but it is very rewarding surgery in such cases to restore vision with minimal complications.

References

1. Tan DT, Janardhanan P, Zhou H, et al. Penetrating keratoplasty in Asian eyes: The Singapore Corneal Transplant Study. *Ophthalmology.* 2008;115:975-982.
2. Pramanik S, Musch DC, Sutphin JE, Farjo AA. Extended long term outcomes of penetrating keratoplasty for keratoconus. *Ophthalmology.* 2006;113:16338.
3. Vajpayee RB, Sharma N, Sinha R, et al. Infectious keratitis following keratoplasty. *Surv Ophthalmol.* 2007;52:1-12.
4. Böhringer D, Sundmacher R, Reinhard T. [Suture complications in penetrating keratoplasty]. *Klin Monbl Augenheilkd.* 2010;227:735-738.
5. Agarwal T, Bandivadekar P, Sharma N, Sagar P, Titiyal JS. Sutureless anterior lamellar keratoplasty with phacoemulsification. *Cornea.* 2015;34(6):615-620.
6. Yeung SN, Lichtinger A, Kim P, Amiran MD, Rootman DS. Retrospective contralateral study comparing deep anterior lamellar keratoplasty with penetrating keratoplasty: a patient's perspective. *Can J Ophthalmol.* 2012;47(4):360-364.
7. Tan DT, Mehta JS. Future directions in lamellar corneal transplantation. *Cornea.* 2007;26(9 suppl 1):S21-S28.
8. Quurke A, Schmidt-Petersen H, Seiler T. Complications in photorefractive keratectomy for myopia correction. *Ophthalmologe.* 1998;95:734-740.
9. Nagy ZZ, Krueger RR, Suveges I. Central bump-like opacity as a complication of high hyperopic photorefractive keratectomy. *Am J Ophthalmol.* 1999;128:636-638.
10. Fogla R, Knyazer B. Microkeratome-assisted two-stage technique of superficial anterior lamellar keratoplasty for Reis-Bücklers corneal dystrophy. *Cornea.* 2014;33(10):1118-1122.
11. Shousha MA, Yoo SH, Kymionis GD, et al. Long-term results of femtosecond laser-assisted sutureless anterior lamellar keratoplasty. *Ophthalmology.* 2011;118(2):315-323.

Please see videos on the accompanying website at
www.healio.com/books/DALKvideos

5

The Big Bubble Technique

Alaa M. Eldanasoury, MD; Sherif Said Tolees, FRCS; and Harkaran S. Bains, BHSc Oph

Anterior lamellar keratoplasty (ALK) involves a partial- or full-thickness resection of the corneal stroma that is replaced by donor tissue. Numerous techniques have been developed for ALK including manual free hand dissection,[1] microkeratome-assisted ALK,[2,3] and deep anterior lamellar keratoplasty (DALK). DALK is a full-thickness, or near–full-thickness, stromal resection down to, or close to, Descemet's membrane (DM). Common indications for DALK include keratoconus and other corneal ectasias, stromal dystrophies, stromal scars and opacities, corneal ulcers, and corneal perforations. Corneal pathologies affecting the endothelium are contraindicated for DALK.

Many techniques[1-10] have been described for DALK, with the ultimate goal in all being to preserve the recipient's healthy endothelium and replace only pathologic stromal tissue. The advantage of this approach includes a significant mitigation of the risk of endothelial rejection and late endothelial failure in cases with stromal pathologies and healthy endothelium. In 1985, Archila[4] described the injection of air above the DM to facilitate the excision of all corneal layers except DM. Sugita and Kondo[5] described fluid dissection to maximize the removal of diseased corneal stroma. Melles[6] described a method to visualize the corneal thickness by filling the anterior chamber with air so that the depth of an instrument relative to the posterior corneal surface was visible during surgery. Jacob[11,12] described her modified technique of pre-Descemetic DALK (PD-DALK) for primary treatment of acute hydrops to avoid scarring and obtain visual, topographic, structural, and biomechanical improvement and decreased dependence on contact lens, while at the same time avoiding comorbidity of 2 surgeries and the risk of scarring over the visual axis necessitating a penetrating keratoplasty (PK).

Jacob S, ed. *Mastering DALK: A Video Textbook on Deep Anterior Lamellar Keratoplasty* (pp 51-66).

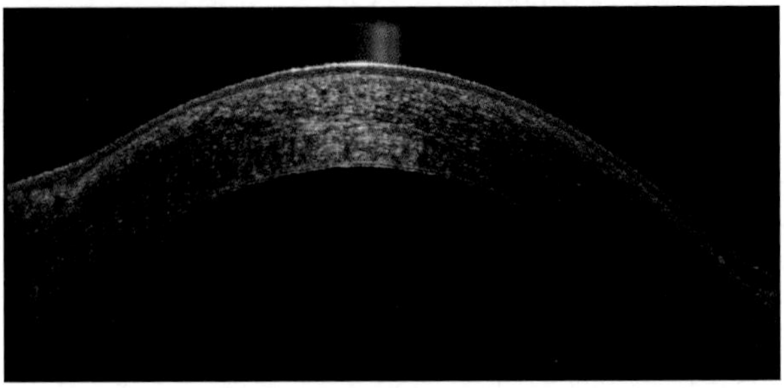

Figure 5-1. Optical coherence tomography (OCT) at 1 year postoperative after D-DALK.

Many modifications in techniques have been published, including viscoelastic dissection,[7] combined air and fluid dissection,[8] and deep parenchyma detachment from the corneal limbus.[9] Anwar and Teichmann[10] described a technique for full dissection of the stroma from DM by injecting a big air bubble in the cleavage plane between DM and the deep stroma inducing a central Descemet's detachment, facilitating complete stromal excision, and reducing the risk of perforation. This technique is called *big bubble DALK*. A recent report[13] of the big bubble technique demonstrated that cleavage takes place between the posterior stroma and a newly described pre-Descemet's layer composed of 5 to 8 collagen lamellae.

Big Bubble DALK

ALK techniques can be divided into 2 main categories based on the depth of dissection: a PD-DALK that leaves variable layers of stroma adherent to DM at the end of the dissection, and the Descemetic procedure (Descemetic DALK [D-DALK]), involving complete stromal excision baring DM or the pre-Descemet's layer (Figure 5-1).

The big bubble technique is the most popular surgical method to obtain a D-DALK,[14] which allows the cleavage separation between DM and posterior stroma by forceful injection of air into the deep stroma. The overall success of this technique in separating the DM from the posterior stroma is approximately 70% to 80% worldwide.[15]

If the big bubble is not obtained, a manual intrastromal dissection has to be performed. The stroma is excised layer-by-layer until the plane of the DM or the pre-Descemetic layer is reached (D-DALK) or a regular deep stromal plane, close to the endothelium is created (PD-DALK)[15,16] (Figure 5-2).

This chapter provides a comprehensive step-by-step description of the big bubble technique for DALK as originally described by Anwar and Teichmann[10] and performed by the authors (over 5000 cases). This chapter guides corneal surgeons who are beginning this procedure or early in their surgical learning curve. The technique described here will highlight the many advantages of DALK with the big bubble technique and surgical pearls are presented for mitigating common difficulties encountered during the learning curve.

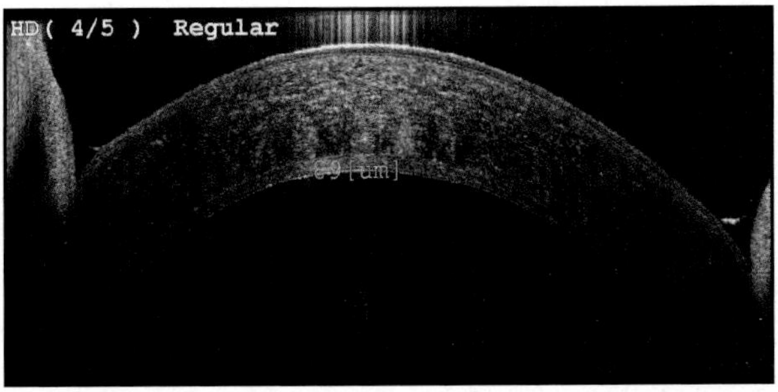

Figure 5-2. OCT at 1 year postoperative after PD-DALK.

Surgical Technique: Step-by-Step Procedure

Recipient Bed Preparation

The patient's eye is prepared and draped in a sterile manner. The center for trephination is marked on the recipient cornea, midway between the geometric center of the cornea and the center of the entrance pupil. The diameter for trephination is chosen to include all or most of the pathologic corneal tissue leaving at least 1.0 mm of clear peripheral recipient cornea for suturing. With a suction trephine, a partial-thickness trephination of the recipient cornea is performed to leave between 50 and 150 μm of corneal thickness. After releasing the suction, the wound is inspected for depth. A depth of approximately 300 μm makes the following steps easier. We prefer the use of a limbal suction trephine with a central obturator because it creates a more vertical trephination wound compared to corneal suction trephines (Figures 5-3 and 5-4 and Video 5-1).

A 27-gauge needle, bent at a 60° angle 4 mm from its tip is introduced bevel down through the bottom of the wound in the central cornea. Many air injection cannulas are commercially available that forego the need to bend needles. The needle has to be in the posterior third of the stroma, which is easy to achieve with an adequate partial trephination. With the needle in place, air is slowly injected into the deep stroma. If the needle is positioned at the proper depth, with more stromal tissue anteriorly than posteriorly, the air will dissect its way between stromal lamellae, creating an area of emphysema before following the path of least resistance, to the anatomic plane between the stroma and pre-Descemet's membrane. This leads to a bullous Descemet detachment, the air bubble in the proper plane can be seen as a well-defined circular bubble raising the central cornea. The big air bubble usually forms between the pre-Descemetic layer and the deep stroma (Type 1 bubble). Less commonly, air dissects its way between the DM and the pre-Descemetic layer (Type 2 bubble). Rarely, 2 bubbles are formed, one in each plane (Type 3 bubble), this is a combination of Type 1 and 2. This is described later in the chapter.

If a big air bubble fails to form and there is relatively high resistance as the air is injected, air will disseminate into the corneal stroma creating surgical emphysema in the superficial corneal tissue. If this occurs, air injection is stopped, the needle withdrawn and reintroduced at a deeper level in an adjacent region of clear cornea. Air

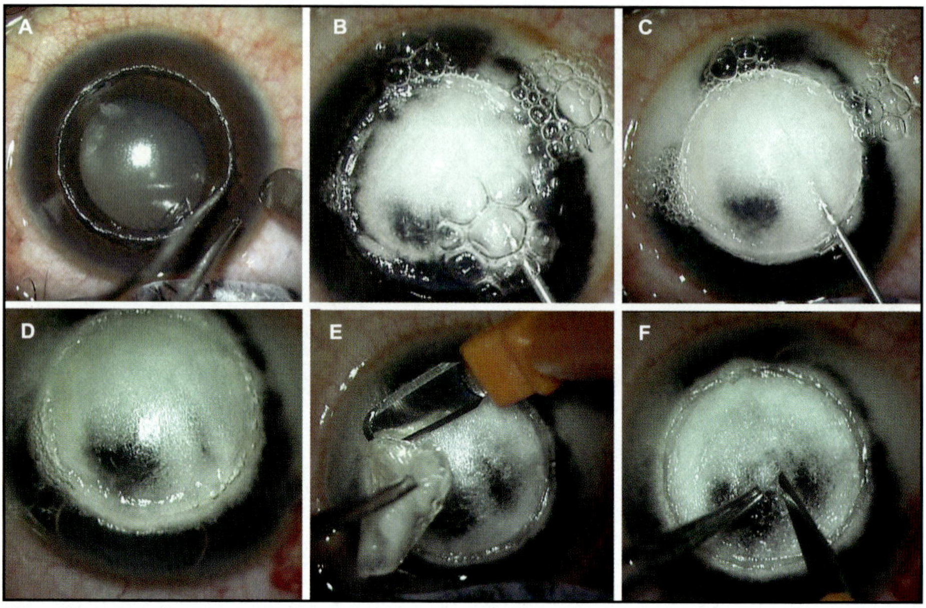

Figure 5-3. Step-by-step procedure. (A) The partially trephined groove on the cornea is deepened with a bevel up crescent blade. (B) A 26-gauge needle is inserted bevel down in the depth of the groove and air injected. The big bubble can be seen expanding. (C) A big bubble is seen formed in the plane between the pre-Descemet's membrane and the Descemetic-endothelial plane. Note the well-defined edge of the bubble. (D) The peripheral bean-shaped configuration acquired by a small air bubble injected in to the anterior chamber confirms the formation of a big bubble. (E) Anterior keratectomy is performed with a blunt crescent blade to remove most of the stromal tissue anterior to the bubble. (F) The air bubble is punctured with a sharp knife with one swift movement to open the big bubble space. (Reprinted with permission from Dr. Soosan Jacob, Dr. Agarwal's Eye Hospital, Chennai, India.)

injection can be repeated until a large bubble is formed or the cornea becomes totally opaque preventing visualization; in this case, an ALK is performed removing opaque stromal tissue and air is injected at a deeper level as described later in the chapter.

Some surgeons described the use of a sharp-tip dissector with a round shaft to facilitate the lamellar dissection by creating a lamellar track for the 27-gauge blunt air injection cannula. According to proponents of this technique, it yields a statistically higher percentage of successful big bubble creation and makes the maneuver more manageable compared to air injection with a needle.[17] In our experience, we did not find a significant difference in the rate of successful bubble creation with the sharp needle vs the use of a dissector and cannula.

Once a big air bubble is obtained, a side port (with a slight vertical orientation to prevent piercing the big bubble) is created in the very peripheral cornea to drain aqueous and lower the pressure in the anterior chamber. Anterior keratectomy is then performed, resecting the anterior portion of the stroma (corneal debulking), this can be easily performed with a round tip blade. At this stage, the large air bubble becomes more evident as the central cornea above the bubble is firm over a soft globe. This is a hallmark that the air bubble is in the correct plane. At this stage the surgeon should

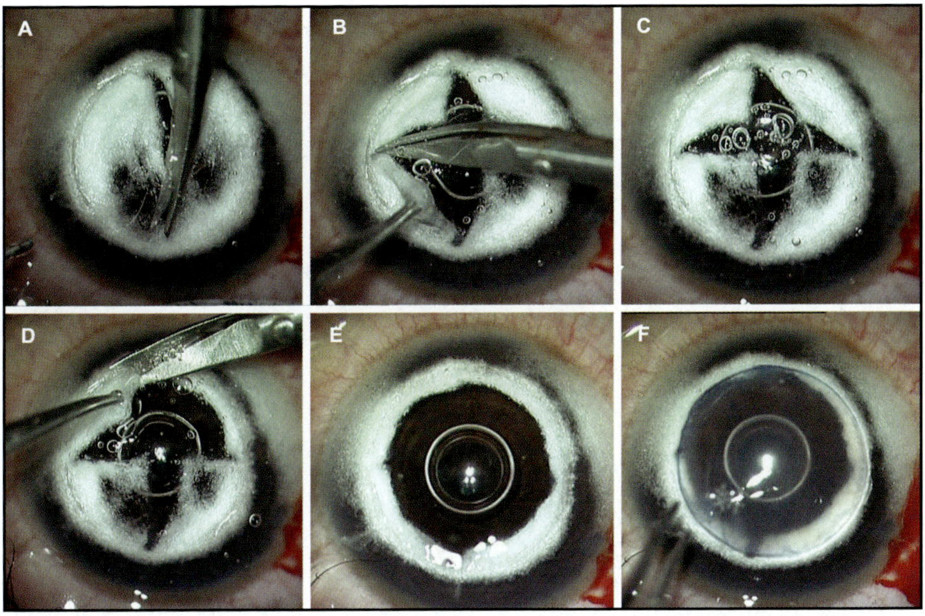

Figure 5-4. Step-by-step procedure (continued). (A-C) Viscoelastic is instilled into the bubble space, and the overlying residual stroma is quadrisected with a Vannas scissors. (D) Residual stromal layer is removed quadrant-wise using blunt-tipped Vannas scissors. (E) Clear pre-Descemet's layer and DM are visualized after stromal dissection with an air bubble in the anterior chamber. (F) The donor graft with DM stripped is sutured on to the host bed. (Reprinted with permission from Dr. Soosan Jacob, Dr. Agarwal's Eye Hospital, Chennai, India.)

also identify the type of bubble formed. Here we describe a typical DALK procedure with the more common Type 1 bubble. Dealing with Type 2 and Type 3 bubbles will be described under the "Surgical Challenges" section later in this chapter.

A sharp knife is used to puncture the bubble, allowing air to escape through the track created by the knife. During air escape, DM can usually be seen slowly moving anteriorly; a surgical descemetocele is then created. A blunt Barraquer spatula (Katena) is introduced through the same track; if the spatula is inserted through the correct track there is no resistance throughout the area dissected by the air bubble. Once the right plane is found, blunt-tip Vannas scissors (Moria) are then used to cut the remaining stromal layers. The scissors blade can be safely introduced in the plane dissected by the air bubble in the area of induced DM separation. The blunt-tip spatula is then used to free the remaining adhesions between the stroma and the DM in the areas not dissected by the bubble. A small pocket can be further dissected past the wound to allow better trimming of the wound edge. Cutting the remaining stroma is usually performed from the center to periphery in 4 quarters. The stromal layer is then removed and the wound edges trimmed to be as vertical as possible to minimize postoperative astigmatism.

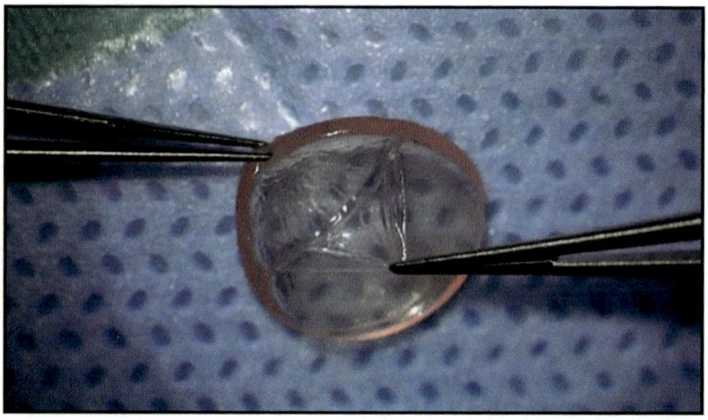

Figure 5-5. DM peeling from the donor tissue using non-toothed forceps.

At this stage, the recipient bed is ready to receive the donor tissue. During dissection, it is advisable to keep the bare DM moist as excessive dryness makes it more brittle and prone to perforation.

Donor Preparation

The donor tissue is cut from the endothelial side using the same diameter blade as used for the recipient. Peeling Descemet and endothelium from the donor tissue can be performed using a dry surgical sponge and/or non-toothed forceps (Figure 5-5). In some cases, the DM with the endothelium can be easily peeled in one layer; this usually occurs with corneal tissue from older donors. In corneal tissue from younger donors (45 years old or younger) DM-endothelium complex can be removed in pieces with a dry sponge. Care should be taken to prevent stromal injury during removal of the endothelium. Watson et al[18] described the use of trypan blue for easier identification of DM and endothelium.

Suturing Donor Graft

The donor tissue is placed over the recipient bed. A 12 or 16 radial marker coated with gentian violet is used to mark both the donor and the recipient tissue, 4 cardinal 10-0 sutures are used to fix the donor in place and 12 or 16 anti-torque running bites are used to secure the donor tissue in place. Suture tension is adjusted based on intraoperative keratoscopy to minimize postoperative astigmatism. Interrupted sutures can be also used according to the surgeon's preference; however, in the authors' experience running sutures are more advantageous for adjusting the tension on the graft intraoperatively as well as during the early postoperative period (Video 5-2).

Postoperative Medications

This includes topical antibiotics and steroids. We prescribe topical antibiotics; Vigamox (moxifloxacillin) until complete closure of the epithelium and topical steroids (Pred forte; prednisolone acetate 1%) 4 times/day for 1 month and then gradually tapered over 6 weeks. We leave the continuous sutures in place for 12 months postoperatively to ensure wound healing and stability. In cases where the sutures become loose or attract blood vessels, they are replaced.

Refractive Rehabilitation

Three months after suture removal, we offer a secondary refractive procedure for cases with high residual refractive errors to decrease spectacle dependence. Secondary refractive procedures include femtosecond-assisted astigmatic keratotomy, laser in situ keratomileusis, and spherical or toric phakic lenses. In our practice, the most common secondary refractive procedure after DALK is toric posterior chamber phakic intraocular lenses.

Surgical Challenges During Big Bubble DALK

During the learning curve, a number of intraoperative challenges can occur. The main challenge is to avoid perforation of DM. The incidence of DM perforation during DALK ranges from 4% to 39.2%[5,8,19-21] and appears to depend on surgeon experience, indications for keratoplasty, and surgical techniques. Keratoconus patients are more prone to DM ruptures than patients with other corneal diseases.[22] Microperforation rates seem to be highest with manual layer-by-layer dissection (26.3%) and lowest with the Anwar big bubble technique (5.48%). Perforation of DM can occur during any step of surgery, including trephination, air injection, stromal excision, and donor suturing.

Perforation During Trephination

If the trephination is too deep and anterior chamber penetration occurs in more than 2 clock hours, completion of the procedure is extremely difficult and conversion to PK is recommended, especially during the learning curve. If a small penetration occurs, the site or penetration can be sutured and big bubble DALK continued by injecting air in a different location distant from the perforation.

Superficial Trephination

Superficial trephination hinders the insertion of the needle at an appropriate depth. In this case deepening of the wound at the needle insertion site can be performed with a sharp knife under direct visualization (Video 5-3).

Descemet's Membrane Perforation Before or During Air Injection

This can occur if the needle is inserted too deeply. In this case, the needle is withdrawn, an air bubble introduced in the anterior chamber through a side port to seal the perforation, and air injection is performed more superficially in a different section of the cornea, and big bubble DALK can still be completed.

Failure of Big Bubble Formation

If a big bubble is not obtained during the initial air injection, the injection can be repeated at a different site; usually 3 or 4 injections can be performed before complete stromal opacification that precludes visualization of the advancing needle. At this stage, anterior keratectomy is performed and air injection is performed again in the remaining deep stroma using a 30-gauge needle (Video 5-4). If the attempted reinjection fails, hydrodelamination or layer-by-layer dissection until DM is exposed can be performed. However, both techniques reduce the chance of exposing DM and increase the risk of perforation.[16]

In some cases where the air bubble is obtained after several attempts, the cornea may be too opaque, precluding the identification of the air bubble. One method to confirm the presence of a bubble is to drain the aqueous from the anterior chamber as the central cornea over the bubble remains firm over a soft eye. A small bubble test can also be performed.[23] This test involves injection of a small air bubble from the paracentesis. If this bubble does not migrate centrally, it indicates the presence of a big bubble occupying the central space in the anterior chamber. This is called the *big bubble small bubble technique.*

Type of Big Bubble Formed

Care must be taken to identify the type of bubble created. Three types of big bubbles can be achieved.[13] A Type 1 big bubble is where the air bubble separates the pre-Descemetic layer from the deep stroma creating a large central bubble of around 8 to 9 mm in diameter. This is the preferred and more common type of bubble in DALK, as the pre-Descemetic layer confers additional strength to the recipient DM-endothelium complex. The less common Type 2 big bubble is where the DM is separated from the posterior surface of pre-Descemetic layer by the air bubble. This big bubble starts forming in the peripheral cornea toward the center, can reach the far periphery of the cornea, and has a thinner wall. Recognition of Type 2 bubble is important as it is more susceptible to tears and bursting; extreme caution is necessary during stromal dissection in these cases (Video 5-5). Type 3 is a mixed big bubble when the previous 2 coexist; usually Type 1 is complete and Type 2 is partial, but both can be complete.[24] For cases with mixed bubble formation, puncture of the Type 1 bubble is recommended and dissection of the stroma above the pre-Descemetic layer is performed. The Type 2 bubble is then evacuated before securing the corneal graft without further dissection at the level of bare DM. In our experience, more than 85% of the big bubbles formed during DALK surgery are Type 1. Type 2 bubbles are less common, and mixed bubble formation is rare.

Formation of a Small Bubble

In DALK surgery, dissection of stroma is much easier if the air bubble is large enough to detach DM from below the central 7 to 8 mm of stroma. In some cases, a small air bubble is formed, and the peripheral stroma not encompassed by the bubble will adhere to DM. At this point, additional air can be injected with a 30-gauge needle in the stroma, close to the small bubble in an effort to enlarge it. This is a technique that we call *bubble augmentation* (Video 5-6). Alternately, separation can be accomplished by blunt dissection with a Barraquer spatula. Of note, once the right plane is achieved stromal separation from DM is invariably easy, even outside the region encompassed by the bubble.

Perforation During Dissection

If microperforation occurs during dissection with the spatula, air can be injected in the anterior chamber to seal the microperforation from within (ie, air tamponade) until the dissection is completed (Video 5-7). Larger perforations that cannot be adequately sealed with an air bubble in the anterior chamber can be sealed with a small piece of stromal tissue (ie, stromal plug). In most cases, this is enough to allow proceeding with the dissection. Large perforations that cannot be sealed with air alone or air with a stromal plug may need sealing with tissue adhesive (ie, fibrin sealant).

Perforation During Suturing

Caution is recommended during suturing to avoid perforation of the DM with the needle. If a perforation occurs, it can be sealed by air injection into the anterior chamber.

Postoperative Complications

The most common early postoperative complication is DM detachment. In most cases, this resolves spontaneously within the first 2 weeks. In the rare cases where a large detachment does not resolve spontaneously, single air injection in the anterior chamber usually suffices to achieve DM attachment. In the last 100 cases performed by the authors, air injection was required once (1%) to reattach DM 3 weeks postoperatively (Figure 5-6).

Stromal rejection although rare, may occur after lamellar keratoplasty (LK).[14,24,25] In our series, the incidence of stromal rejection after DALK was less than 6%. Stromal rejection usually responds well to topical steroids and resolves in most cases. Cases of stromal rejection unresponsive to medical treatment may end in corneal scarring and vascularization. In these cases a regraft is required, and it is possible to replace the full-thickness corneal stroma and preserve the recipient endothelium. This is an important advantage of DALK with exposure of DM. However, in cases with near Descemet dissection, where the DM is not exposed in the primary surgery,

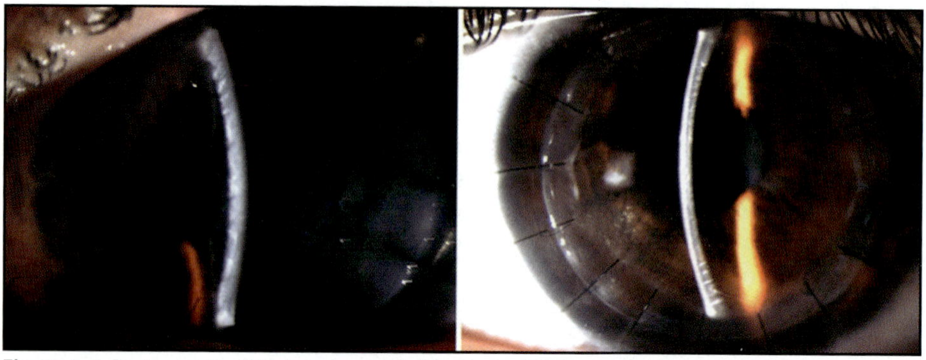

Figure 5-6. Postoperative DM detachment (left); attached DM post–air injection (right).

Figure 5-7. Inflammatory necrosis of the graft.

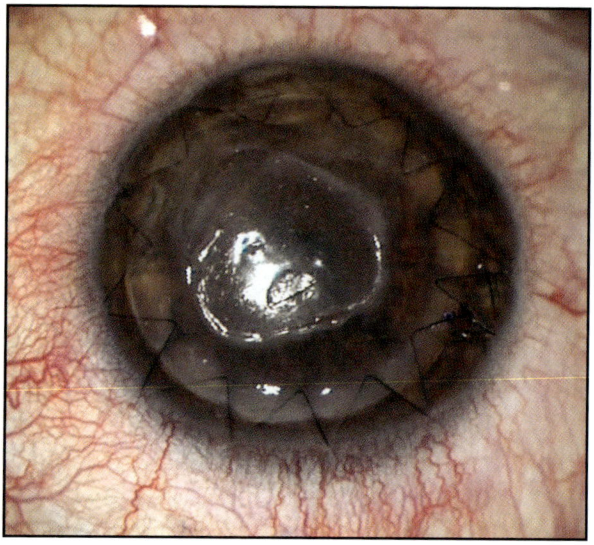

regrafting while preserving the DM may be difficult as the interface can be scarred and vascularized.

Inflammatory necrosis of the graft is a very rare complication of unknown etiology (< 1/1000 cases, in our experience; Figure 5-7). It has also been described in cases of penetrating keratoplasty, where the graft shows signs of sterile inflammation and no immunologic causes were detected.[26]

Clinical Outcomes

We conducted a prospective study of 105 eyes of 105 consecutive patients with moderate or advanced keratoconus scheduled for DALK at the Magrabi Eye and Ear Hospital, Jeddah, Saudi Arabia. Follow-up rates over time were:

- 92 (87.6%) eyes at 1 month
- 80 (76.2%) eyes at 3 months
- 84 (80%) eyes at 6 months
- 99 (94.3%) eyes at 12 months
- 88 (83.8%) eyes at 18 months

All surgeries were performed by 1 surgeon (AME). Sixty-eight (68.7%) eyes had their sutures removed after 12 months examination.

Reproducibility of the Surgical Procedure

Successful separation of DM with the big bubble technique was performed in 95/105 (90.5%) eyes. Of these eyes, DM was successfully separated with a big bubble at the first injection in 77 (73.3%) eyes; 11 (10.5%) eyes at the second injection; 6 (5.7%) eyes at the third injection; and 1 (1.0%) eye at the fifth injection. The big bubble formation failed in 10 (9.5%) eyes.

Descemet exposure was achieved in 100 (95.2%) eyes and near Descemet dissection in 5 (4.8%) eyes. In the eyes with near Descemet dissection, 4 (3.8%) eyes had unsuccessful bubble formation and 1 (0.95%) eye experienced early air escape during anterior keratectomy after successful bubble formation.

Visual Outcomes

Mean uncorrected-distance visual acuity increased from 1.37 (20/400) preoperatively to 0.57 (20/80) postoperatively.

Mean corrected-distance visual acuity (CDVA) was 0.84 (20/125) in the group of 73 eyes that could be refracted preoperatively. At 1 year postoperatively, the mean CDVA was 0.15 (20/27) in the same group.

There were no significant differences between the postoperative CDVA of eyes that could be refracted and eyes that could not be refracted preoperatively (due to high corneal irregularity).

Preoperatively, CDVA was 0.3 (20/32) in 9 (8.6%) eyes and 0.4 (20/50) or worse in 96 (91.4%) eyes. At 12 months, CDVA was 0.0 (20/20) or better in 31 (31.3%) eyes, 0.2 (20/32) or better in 81 (81.8%) eyes and 0.3 (20/40) or better in 87 (87.9%) eyes and 0.4 (20/50) or worse in 12 (12.1%) eyes. No eyes lost 1 or more lines of CDVA at 1 year postoperatively and 96% eyes gained one or more lines, 82% gained 3 or more lines, and 50% gained more than 5 lines.

Refractive Outcomes

Preoperatively, the mean refractive spherical equivalent (MRSE) was -5.59 ± 5.96 diopters (D) (range: -20.75 to 4.00 D) in the 73 eyes that could be refracted. One year after DALK, the mean (MRSE) was -1.58 ± 3.32 D (range: -19.25 to 4.38 D) in 100 eyes. Preoperatively, the mean refractive cylinder was -6.90 ± 2.39 D (range: 0.00 to -13.00 D) in 73 eyes; 1 year after DALK, the mean refractive cylinder was -3.88 ± 2.26 D (range: 0.00 to -10.00 D) in 100 eyes.

Topographic Analysis

Preoperatively, 87 (82.9%) eyes had valid corneal topographies examinations. Corneal topography was available in 82 (78%) eyes at 12 months postoperatively and in 82 (78%) eyes at 18 months postoperatively.

Data from the OPD Scan III (Nidek Co. Ltd.) were used to analyze the change in simulated keratometry (simK), average pupillary power, average corneal power, corneal cylinder, surface regularity index (SRI), and surface asymmetry index (SAI). SRI and SAI are the optimal indices for describing surface regularity and symmetry.

The change in corneal high-order wavefront root mean square, horizontal and vertical coma, and corneal asphericity were also analyzed using the OPD Scan III.

All indices improved statistically significantly between preoperatively and 12 months postoperatively ($P < 0.05$, all cases). The mean root mean square of the total corneal high-order aberrations in all eyes decreased statistically significantly at 12 and 18 months postoperatively compared to preoperatively ($P = .00$ and $P = .00$, respectively; Table 5-1).

Most corneal indices showed a significant improvement after DALK. Preoperatively, the mean SRI was 1.89 ± 0.29 (range: 1.29 to 2.9) and SAI was 1.88 ± 1.17 (range: 1.2 to 7.49); 1 year after DALK, both indices decreased significantly to 1.3 ± 0.25 (range: 0.6 to 1.93) and 1.18 ± 0.25 (range: 0.57 to 1.75), respectively. This improvement reflects the better quality of vision after DALK.

Suture Removal

We routinely keep DALK sutures in place for 1 year postoperatively to allow for wound stabilization and to decrease the effect of suture removal on corneal shape. Indications for suture removal after 1 year include astigmatism greater than 3.00 D, anisometropia, and unwillingness or inability to tolerate prescription glasses to correct ametropia. If the patient is satisfied with his or her CDVA, we keep the sutures in place and instruct the patient to present for examination every 6 months. We evaluated 59 eyes that completed both the 12-month examination (before suture removal) and the 18-month examination (at least 3 months after suture removal). In this group of eyes, MRSE changed from -1.58 D (range: -19.25 to 4.00 D) before removal to -1.47 D (range: -10.00 to 5.00 D) after suture removal. The mean refractive cylinder at 12 months was -4.36 ± 2.3 D and -4.90 ± 2.9 D at 18 months. The mean change in refractive cylinder in the 59 eyes was 1.92 ± 1.67 D (range: 0.00 to 7.00 D) after suture removal.

The refractive cylinder decreased between 1.1 and 3.5 D in 14 (23.7%) eyes. The refractive cylinder increased by 1.1 to 3.5 D in 12 (20.3%) eyes, and between 3.6 and 7.0 D in 9 (15.3%) eyes. The double-angle refractive cylinder vector change indicated unpredictable changes in cylinder after suture removal.

Table 5-1

Topographic Indices and Corneal Wavefront of Eyes With Moderate and Advanced Keratoconus Before and After DALK With the Big Bubble Technique

	ACP	CYL	DSI	SRI	SAI	OSI	Q Value	Corneal Total HO RMS	Corneal SA (C12)
Before DALK									
N	87	87	87	87	87	86	80	80	88
Average	55.08	7.88	16.29	1.89	1.88	13.00	-1.51	3.59	-0.88
Standard Deviation	7.14	4.10	6.39	0.29	1.17	5.89	1.86	1.66	0.97
Minimum	32.69	0.70	5.84	1.29	1.20	2.61	-4.83	0.48	-4.23
Maximum	72.34	20.94	35.51	2.90	7.49	30.97	8.35	9.05	1.66
12 Months After DALK									
N	82	82	82	82	82	82	82	82	77
Average	44.03	4.12	6.60	1.30	1.18	4.32	-0.75	1.14	-0.11
Standard Deviation	1.95	2.03	2.63	0.25	0.25	2.58	0.86	0.52	0.34
Minimum	39.53	0.26	2.02	0.60	0.57	0.95	-3.50	0.44	-1.06
Maximum	49.38	8.19	12.79	1.93	1.75	10.89	1.17	2.95	0.54

(continued)

Table 5-1 (continued)

Topographic Indices and Corneal Wavefront of Eyes With Moderate and Advanced Keratoconus Before and After DALK With the Big Bubble Technique

	ACP	CYL	DSI	SRI	SAI	OSI	Q Value	Corneal Total HO RMS	Corneal SA (C12)
18 Months After DALK									
N	82	82	82	82	82	82	82	79	77
Average	43.93	4.08	6.35	1.20	1.05	3.93	-0.15	1.27	0.13
Standard Deviation	2.01	2.47	2.17	0.27	0.21	1.88	0.79	0.62	0.30
Minimum	40.20	0.31	1.57	0.52	0.53	0.57	-2.80	0.51	-0.86
Maximum	50.49	11.91	11.06	1.82	1.51	9.36	1.65	3.18	0.85
18 Months After DALK (Suture-Out)									
N	56	56	56	56	56	56	56	52	52
Average	44.25	4.66	6.35	1.23	1.06	3.75	0.08	1.35	0.22
Standard Deviation	2.11	2.55	1.93	0.27	0.20	1.57	0.61	0.68	0.23
Minimum	40.20	0.52	1.57	0.68	0.61	0.57	-0.94	0.51	-0.20
Maximum	50.49	11.91	9.94	1.82	1.51	7.29	1.65	3.18	0.85

ACP = mean corneal power at 5.0 mm; C12 = corneal spherical aberration; CYL = topographic cylinder; DSI = differential sectorial index; HO = high order aberration; OSI = opposite sector index; RMS = root mean square; Q value = asphericity value.

All corneal aberrations are measured at 5 mm and to the 6th order. Suture-in indicates eyes with retained sutures; suture-out indicates eyes that fulfilled the criteria for postoperative suture removal and the sutures were removed.

Advantages and Disadvantages of Big Bubble DALK

The advantage of the big bubble technique is that a wide surface area of DM may be readily exposed with fewer risks of perforation compared to other manual stromal dissection techniques. Furthermore, this procedure may be employed in patients with very ectatic and thinned corneas, where other manual stromal dissection techniques may be unsafe.

Compared to manual stromal dissection,[1] and microkeratome-assisted LK,[2,3] D-DALK with baring of the DM has the advantage of better visual outcome because of the better optical quality due to the absence of interface healing and possible haze or scarring. Soong et al[27] and Saini et al[1] reported that graft-host interface opacification and/or vascularization were the most common vision-limiting factors after conventional LK. In a retrospective study comparing D-DALK with PK in patients with keratoconus, Watson et al[18] found no significant difference in final CDVA between both groups; they also reported no significant difference in postoperative astigmatism 28 months after surgery.

A disadvantage of the big bubble technique is that frequency of successful air bubble formation depends on surgeon experience.

A limitation of this technique is the presence of deep corneal scarring involving DM or previous perforation. In these cases, when air is injected, direct passage of air into the anterior chamber is often observed as a result of DM interruption. It may therefore be advisable to try to avoid Descemetic scarring secondary to conventional management of acute hydrops by employing the Jacob modified technique for acute hydrops[11,12] that is described in detail elsewhere in this book.

References

1. Saini JS, Jain AK, Sukhija J, Saroha V. Indications and outcome of optical partial thickness lamellar keratoplasty. *Cornea*. 2003;22(2):111-113.
2. Tan DT, Ang LP. Automated lamellar therapeutic keratoplasty for post-PRK corneal scarring and thinning. *Am J Ophthalmol*. 2004;136:1067-1069.
3. Busin M, Zambianchi L, Arffa RC. Microkeratome-assisted lamellar keratoplasty for the surgical treatment of keratoconus. *Ophthalmology*. 2005;112(6):987-997.
4. Archila EA. Deep lamellar keratoplasty for dissection of host tissue with intrastromal air injection. *Cornea*. 1984;3:217-218.
5. Sugita J, Kondo J. Deep lamellar keratoplasty with complete removal of pathological stroma for vision improvement. *Br J Ophthalmol*. 1997;81:184-188.
6. Melles GR, Lander F, Rietveld F, et al. A new surgical technique for deep stromal, anterior lamellar keratoplasty. *Br J Ophthalmol*. 1999;83:327-333.
7. Manche EE, Holland GN, Maloney RK. Deep lamellar keratoplasty using viscoelastic dissection. *Arc Ophthalmol*. 1999;117:1561-1565.
8. Tsubota K, Kaido M, Yu M, et al. A new surgical technique for deep lamellar keratoplasty with single running suture adjustment. *Am J Ophthalmol*. 1998;126:1-8.
9. Senoo T, Chiba K, Terada O, et al. Deep lamellar keratoplasty by deep parenchyma detachment from the corneal limbus. *Br J Ophthalmol*. 2005;89;1597-1600.

10. Anwar M, Teichmann KD. Deep lamellar keratoplasty. Surgical techniques for anterior lamellar keratoplasty with and without baring of Descemet's membrane. *Cornea.* 2002;21:374-383.
11. Jacob S, Narasimhan S, Agarwal A, Sambath J, Umamaheshwari G, Saijimol AI. Primary modified predescemetic deep anterior lamellar keratoplasty in acute corneal hydrops. *Cornea.* 2018;37(10):1328-1333.
12. Jacob S. Primary predescemetic DALK for acute hydrops Soosan Jacob with audio [video]. YouTube. https://www.youtube.com/watch?v=5ZeAXOmVDJw. Published June 14, 2018. Accessed September 27, 2018.
13. Dua HS, Faraj LA, Said DG, Gray T, Lowe J. Human corneal anatomy redefined: a novel pre-Descemet's layer (Dua's layer). *Ophthalmology.* 2013;120(9):1778–1785.
14. Anwar M, Teichmann KD. Big-bubble technique to bare DM in anterior lamellar keratoplasty. *J Cataract Refract Surg.* 2002;28(3):398-403.
15. Reinhart WJ, Musch DC, Jacobs DS, Lee WB, Kaufman SC, Shtein RM. Deep anterior lamellar keratoplasty as an alternative to penetrating keratoplasty: a report by the American Academy of Ophthalmology. *Ophthalmology.* 2011;118(1):209-218.
16. Sarnicola V, Toro P, Gentile D, Hannush SB. Descemetic DALK and predescemetic DALK: outcomes in 236 cases of keratoconus. *Cornea.* 2010;29(1):53-59.
17. Sarnicola E, Sarnicola C, Sabatino F, Tosi GM, Perri P, Sarnicola V. Cannula DALK versus needle DALK for keratoconus. *Cornea.* 2016;35(12):1508-1511.
18. Watson SL, Ramsay A, Dart JKG, et al. Comparison of deep lamellar keratoplasty and penetrating keratoplasty in patients with keratoconus. *Ophthalmology.* 2004;111:1676-1682.
19. Fogla R, Padmanabham P. Results of deep lamellar keratoplasty using the big-bubble technique in patients with keratoconus. *Am J Ophthalmol.* 2006;141:254-259.
20. Coombes AG, Kirwan JF, Rostron CK. Deep lamellar keratoplasty with lyophilised tissue in the management of keratoconus. *Br J Ophthalmol.* 2001;85:788-791.
21. Melles GR, Remeijer L, Geerards AJ, Beekhuis WH. The future of lamellar keratoplasty. *Curr Opin Ophthalmol.* 1999;10:253-259.
22. Shimmura S, Shimazaki J, Omoto M, Teruya A, Ishioka M, Tsubota K. Deep lamellar keratoplasty (DLKP) in keratoconus patients using viscoadaptive viscoelastics. *Cornea.* 2005;24:178-181.
23. Fontana L, Parente G, Tassinari G. Simple test to confirm cleavage with air between Descemet's membrane and stroma during big-bubble deep anterior lamellar keratoplasty. *J Cataract Refract Surg.* 2007;33(4):570-572.
24. Dua HS,Katamish T, Said DG, Faraj LA. Differentiating type 1 from type 2 big bubbles in deep anterior lamellar keratoplasty. *Clin Ophthalmol.* 2015;9:1155-1157.
25. Abdelkader A, Kaufman HE. Descemetic versus predescemetic lamellar keratoplasty: clinical and confocal study. *Cornea.* 2011;30(11):1244-1252.
26. American Academy of Ophthalmology. Clinical approach to corneal transplantation. In: *External Disease and Cornea.* San Francisco, CA: American Academy of Ophthalmology; 2017.
27. Soong HK, Katz DJ, Farjo AA, et al. Central lamellar keratoplasty for optical indications. *Cornea.* 1999;18:249-256.

Please see videos on the accompanying website at
www.healio.com/books/DALKvideos

6

Pre-Descemetic DALK

Rishi Swarup, FRCS and T. Suchi Smitha, MS, DNB, FCRS

Deep anterior lamellar keratoplasty (DALK) aims at retaining the host Descemet's membrane (DM) and endothelium while removing the stromal layers completely or near completely wherever possible. Among the various techniques described for DALK, the big bubble technique achieves complete removal of stromal fibers and gives a Descemetic DALK (D-DALK), which is considered ideal, as visual results of D-DALK are comparable to penetrating keratoplasty (PK).[1] Nearly all other methods described for DALK may retain deep stromal fibers to a varying extent, leading to a pre Dua's or pre-Descemetic DALK (PD-DALK), or a near-Descemetic DALK (Figure 6-1).

The level of dissection by the surgeon often depends on the indication for surgery, expertise of the surgeon, and preexisting scar or breach in DM (where the surgeon chooses to retain deeper layers of stroma to prevent perforation of DM, thus avoiding conversion of the procedure to full-thickness keratoplasty). The main concern regarding D-DALK is the unpredictability of the surgical procedure, especially in the hands of a novice surgeon, perforation of DM being the main concern.[2] In case perforation occurs, even if a lamellar procedure can be completed, it may sometimes lead to a low-quality corneal bed. Also, at times, a donor cornea with good quality endothelium may not be available, in the event the procedure needs to be converted to a PK. PD-DALK may have a higher chance of safety against perforation of DM compared to D-DALK, especially in situations where there is a possible weakness in DM or in the hands of a less-experienced surgeon.

Though earlier studies have shown anterior lamellar keratoplasty (ALK) to be inferior to PK as far as visual results are concerned, with regards to PD-DALK, there

Jacob S, ed. *Mastering DALK: A Video Textbook on Deep Anterior Lamellar Keratoplasty* (pp 67-79).

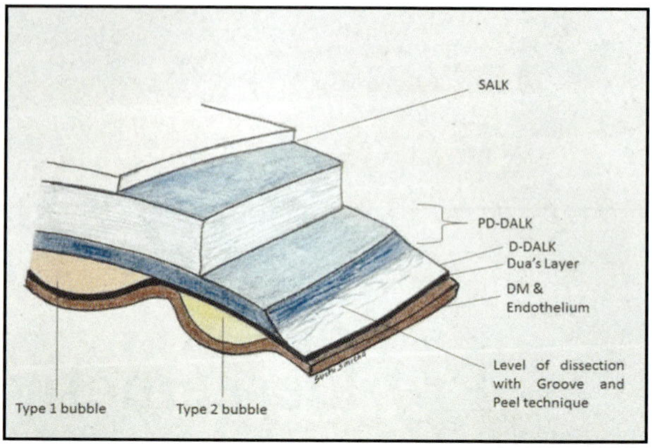

Figure 6-1. Illustration showing levels of dissection in various forms of ALK and potential spaces for bubble formation during DALK. (SALK=superficial anterior lamellar keratoplasty.)

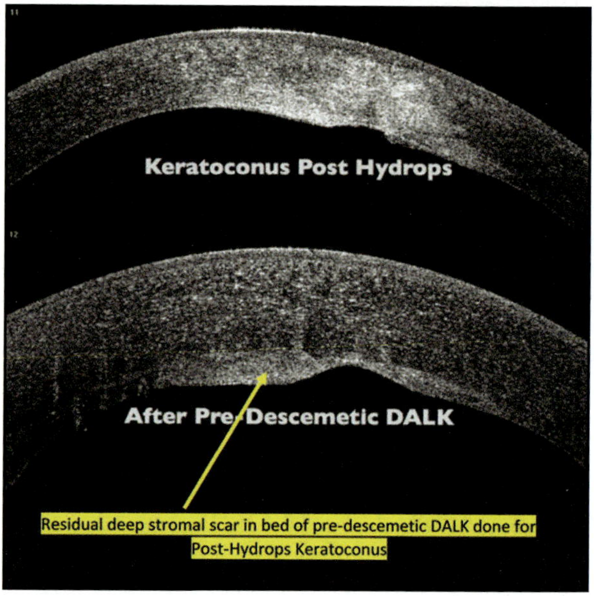

Figure 6-2. Optical coherence tomography (OCT) of PD-DALK done for a case of post-hydrops keratoconus. Small microperforation resulted in some unplanned stromal tissue being left residually in the central bed.

is some evidence at present to show that if the rear stroma is healthy, and if very little stroma is left behind during dissection, it may not hamper the final visual outcome.[3] Thus, intentional sparing of the deepest stromal layers could be considered in order to prevent intraoperative DM rupture in selected cases where DM baring is difficult (Figures 6-2 and 6-3).

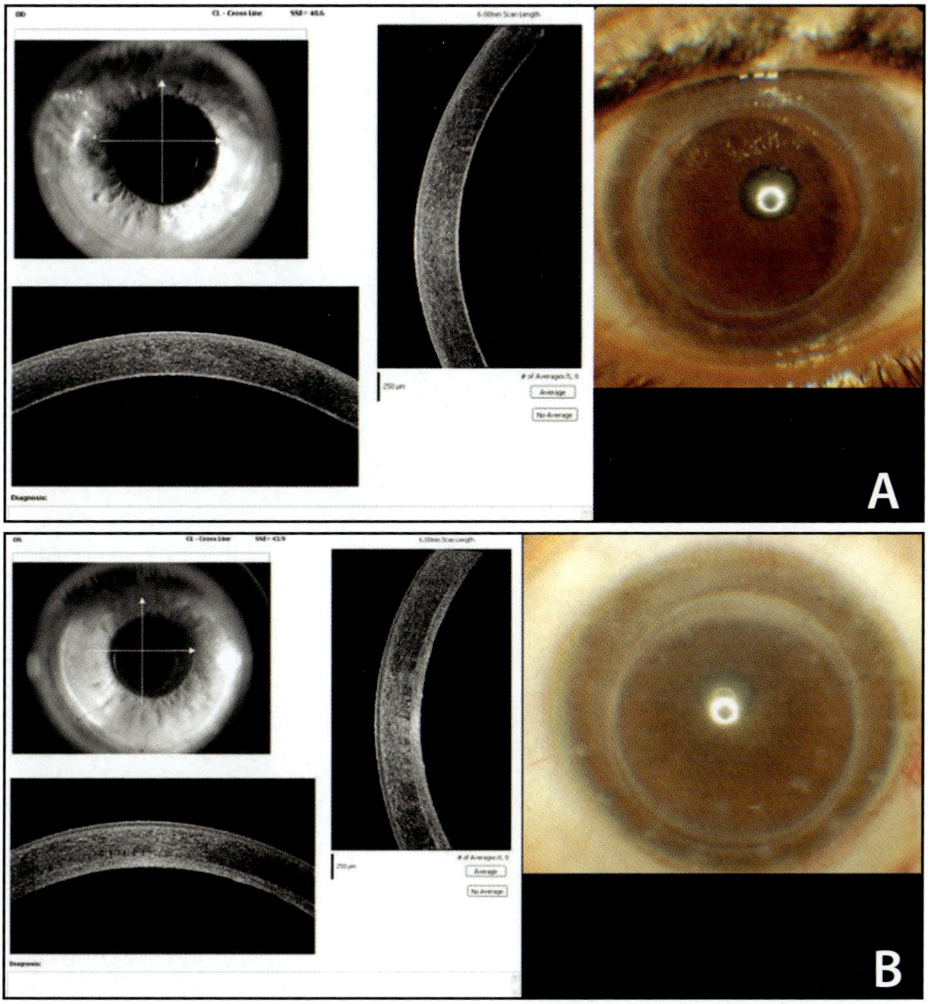

Figure 6-3. (A) Descemetic big bubble DALK of right eye of a patient with macular dystrophy showing a clear graft on the clinical photograph and well-apposed interface on OCT. (B) PD-DALK done for left eye of macular dystrophy case in A showing hyper-reflective stromal bed on OCT with mild graft haze on clinical photograph.

Indications for Pre-Descemetic DALK

Specific indications for PD-DALK include keratoconus eyes that have had previous hydrops, eyes with traumatic penetrating injuries to the central cornea, or severe microbial infections with residual scarring close to DM,[4] iatrogenic ectasia post-keratotomy with deep cuts,[5] and cases where the big bubble technique of DALK should be avoided to prevent perforation of DM (Figures 6-4 and 6-5). It may also be done for acute hydrops using the Jacob modified technique[6,7] as described in detail elsewhere in this book.

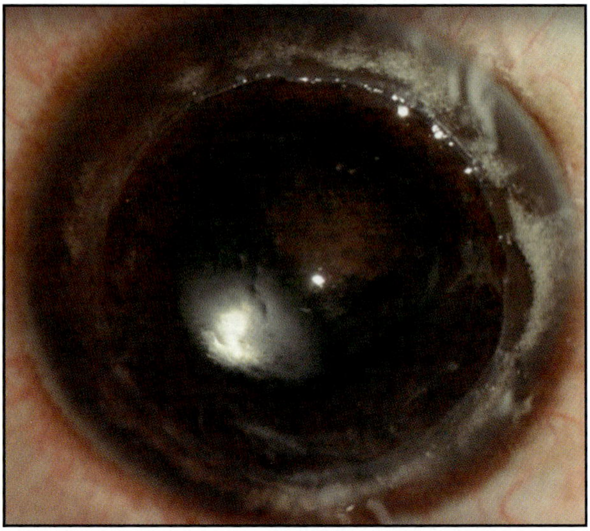

Figure 6-4. Mild residual stromal tissue after excising stromal tissue in PD-DALK.

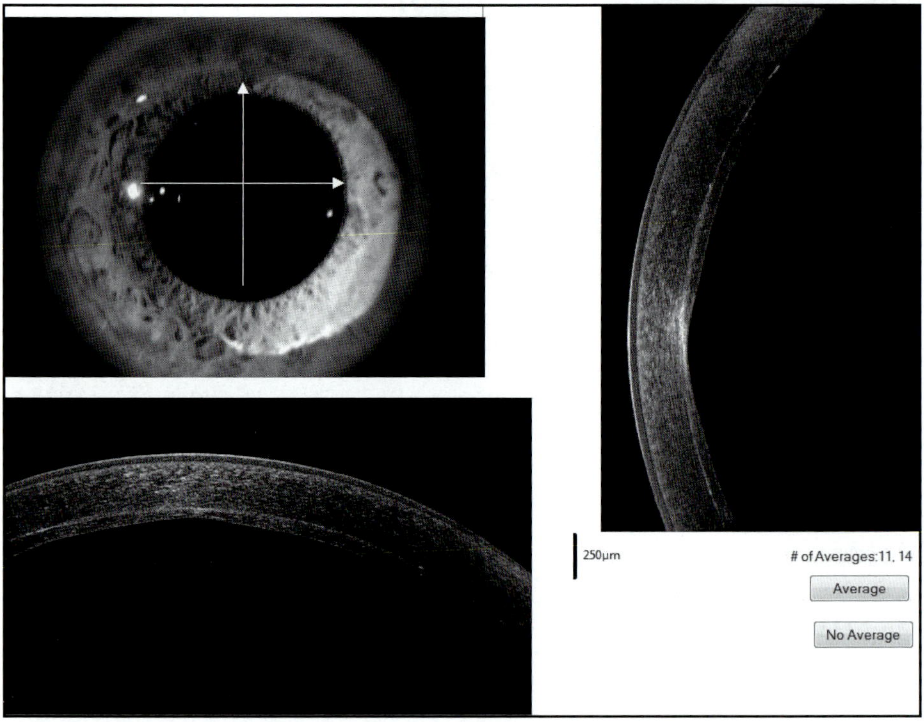

Figure 6-5. Postoperative OCT showing uneven stromal bed with interface hyper-reflectivity in a case of manual PD-DALK.

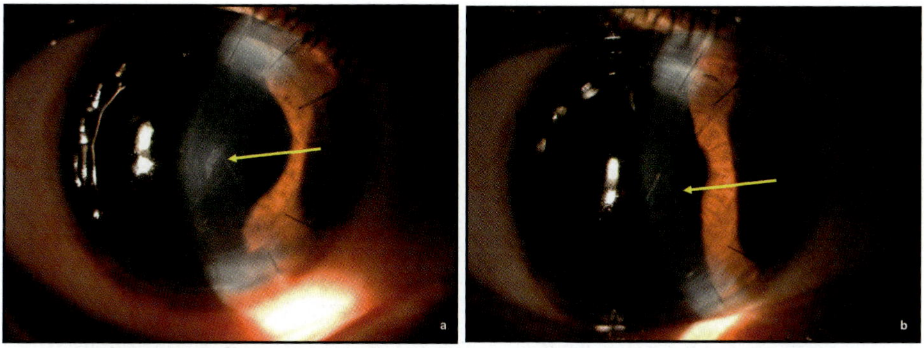

Figure 6-6. (A, B) DALK microperforation during manual DALK, salvaged with air bubble.

Surgical Technique of Pre-Descemetic DALK

Where possible, the surgeon should aim for a D-DALK (ie, to bare the Dua's layer ideally at least in the visual axis). The most accepted technique of D-DALK is currently the big bubble technique, invented by Anwar and Teichmann[8,9]; however, in this technique, if the surgeon fails to obtain a big bubble he or she may choose to dissect layer-by-layer to reach as close as possible to DM. Due to the presence of thin stromal support for the DM, the chances of salvaging a PD-DALK may be better than D-DALK in the event of perforation of DM during dissection, and the thin stromal support can often prevent a microperforation from becoming a macroperforation[10] (Figure 6-6).

If sharp dissectors are used as in Conventional Manual (Cut and Peel) DALK, which involves layer-by-layer excision of the stroma until the desired depth is reached, there may be a higher risk of perforation from the dissectors.

The Melles technique of PD-DALK (described elsewhere in detail in this book), involving utilization of the air-endothelial reflex and introduction of curved dissectors in the deep stroma, may be safer, but can give suboptimal results due to higher possibility of interface scarring between host stromal bed and donor stromal button.[8]

In case a PD-DALK is primarily planned, during initial dissection, use of a diamond knife with calibration set at 50 µm less than thinnest corneal pachymetry has been described, in order to spare a thin deep stromal layer along with DM and endothelium. Subsequently, the pocket created at the desired depth can be enlarged with dissectors to get the right plane. Viscoelastic may be used in aiding dissection.[11]

The Groove and Peel technique[12] is yet another safe technique of achieving a near D-DALK and overcomes many of these difficulties without the need for expensive instrumentation or tremendous surgical skill, making it the ideal technique for the novice lamellar surgeon (Figures 6-7 and 6-8). It involves partial-thickness trephination of the cornea using a simple or guarded trephine until about 50% to 75% depth. At one point in the trephination groove, the groove is slightly deepened using a Bard Parker blade (Aspen Surgical) to create a stromal pocket. Blunt-tipped curved corneal scissors are introduced into this pocket with the blades of the scissors oriented horizontally and the tips closed. Once the tips are intrastromal, the blades are slowly

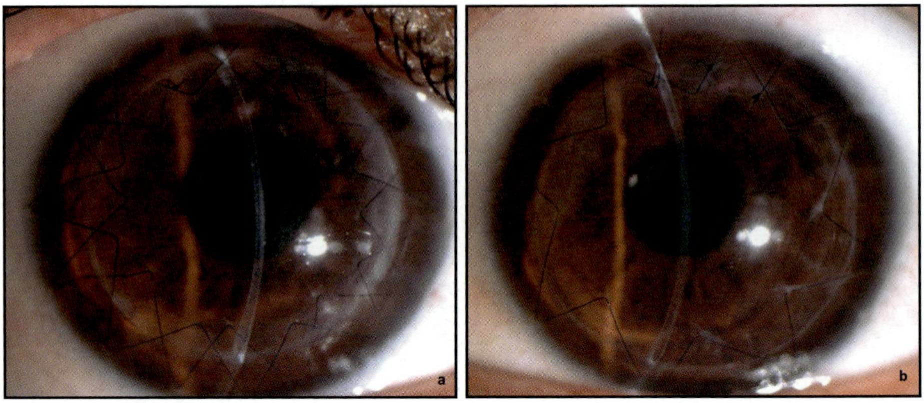

Figure 6-7. Postoperative clinical photographs of right and left eyes of a same patient. (A) Right eye underwent Groove and Peel DALK whereas (B) left eye underwent big bubble DALK, both showing equally clear grafts with clean interface.

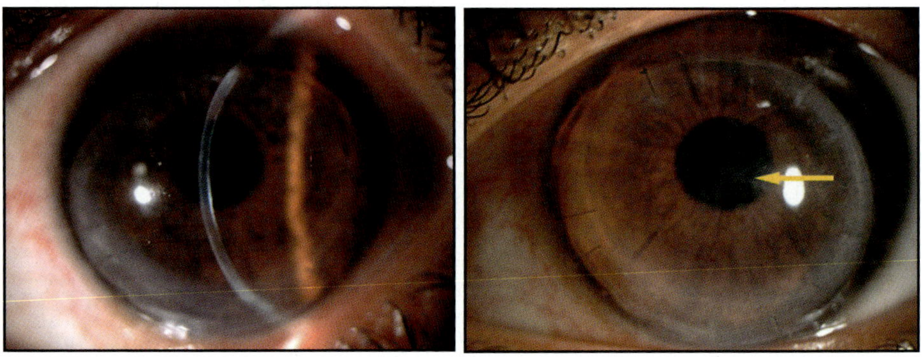

Figure 6-8. (A, B) One-year postoperative clinical photograph of patient in Figure 6-2 showing mild interface scarring at the site of residual scar tissue. Best spectacle-corrected visual acuity at 1 year was 20/30.

opened to separate the collagen lamellae and, hence, widen the intrastromal pocket (Figures 6-9 through 6-11). The anterior layer of this pocket is cut with the scissors and the dissection is advanced in a similar manner along the trephination groove. This blunt dissection is slowly progressed along the entire length of the trephination mark until a circular stromal gutter is created. As the dissection proceeds from one end to the other, the plane of separation gradually advances deeper in the stroma in a spiraling fashion with each pass such that one may complete 2 or 3 turns of the spiral before the desired depth is achieved. This spiraling dissection is to be halted once the Dua's layer is visualized, seen as a glistening clear membrane devoid of any significant overlying stromal attachments. At this point, making a paracentesis, helps to decompress the anterior chamber and reduces the chances of DM perforation. Once the correct plane is reached, the dissection is free of any resistance and the exposure of Dua's layer is slowly increased until 3 to 4 clock hours. The stromal edge is then grasped and tented up (see Figures 6-9, 6-11, and 6-12). Stretch forces, thus

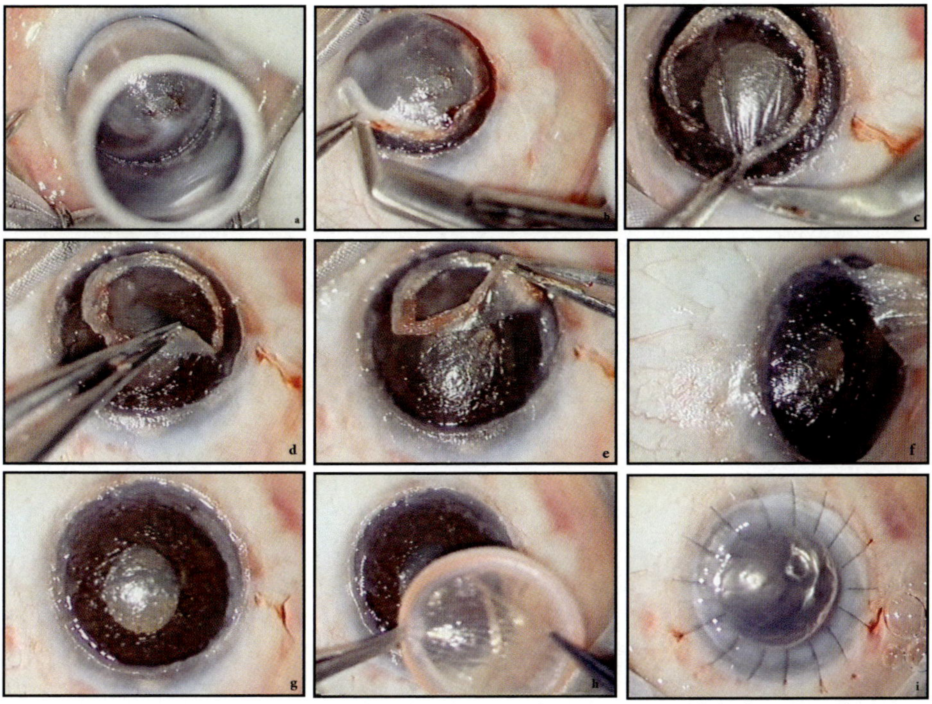

Figure 6-9. Surgical steps: Groove and Peel technique of DALK. (A) Partial-thickness trephination. (B) Creation of initial gutter. (C) Spiral groove until DM is reached. (D) Stromal tissue grasped and tented up under traction. (E) Stretch forces are distributed over a large surface area of the DM. (F) Entire stroma is peeled off in one smooth sweeping motion. (G) Prepared host bed with bare DM;. (H) Donor corneal button is denuded of DM and endothelium. (I) Stromal button sutured in place with interrupted 10-0 nylon sutures.

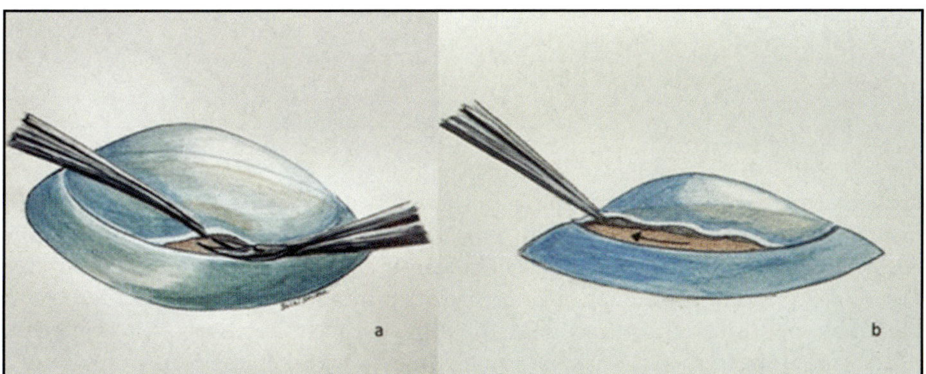

Figure 6-10. Groove and Peel technique of DALK. (A) Expanding the initial pocket made in deep stroma using blunt scissors after partial-thickness trephination. (B) Spiral dissection of the plane to reach the DM in the periphery.

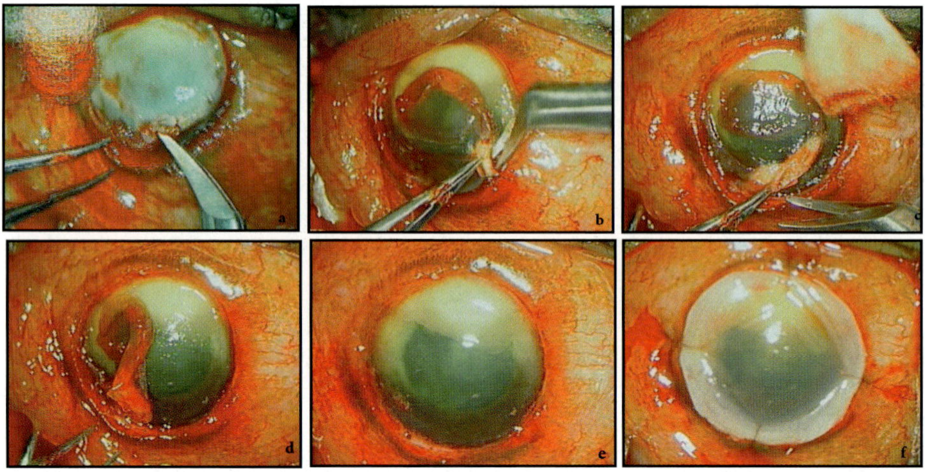

Figure 6-11. Groove and Peel DALK in acanthamoeba keratitis. (A) Partial-thickness trephination encompassing the entire infiltrated stroma. (B) Creation of a spiraling groove all around after excising a layer of stroma to facilitate visualization. (C) The spiral dissection proceed deeper until the pre-Descemet's space is reached. (D) Stromal tissue is grasped and peeled away under traction. (E) Bare DM with an underlying fixed hypopyon in the anterior chamber. (F) Stromal bed is placed in host bed and sutured with 10-0 nylon.

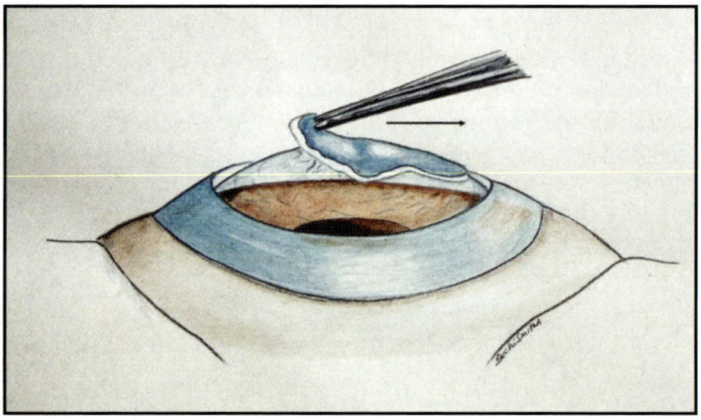

Figure 6-12. Tenting up stromal tissue and peeling the stromal layers from underlying DM in such a way that tension forces are distributed over a larger area in Groove and Peel technique of DALK.

created, help cleave the microscopic adhesions between the deep stroma and DM. In one continuous motion, the entire stroma within the trephination groove is easily peeled away using traction forces distributed over a large surface area of the DM (see Figure 6-9F). Counter-traction may be provided by means of a fixation forceps at the limbus opposite to the direction of the applied force. A relatively easy peeling off of the stroma from the DM has been noted in eyes with keratoglobus (unpublished observation), thus making this technique possibly very predictable and simpler in such cases and where the cornea has become extremely thinned out.

Once the host dissection has been completed, the donor corneal button is trephined to appropriate size. The anterior edge of this button is then grasped with toothed forceps and the endothelial edge dried with a surgical sponge gently rubbing the inner edge of the button with the tip of the sponge. This maneuver makes the DM edge stand up distinctly. This edge is then grasped with non-toothed forceps, such as suture tying forceps, and slowly peeled away from the underside of the corneal button. Trypan blue may be used to visualize and completely remove the host DM. The stromal button is then placed in the host bed and sutured with interrupted/continuous 10-0 nylon sutures[8] (see Figure 6-9).

Intraoperative optical coherence tomography (iOCT) is yet another method that has been described in recent times to visualize dissection depth and various steps in DALK.[13,14] An iOCT helps guide the pre-Descemetic dissection, preventing perforation or leaving behind an irregularly thick bed.[15]

Though Femtosecond laser is also a tool tried for DALK,[16] it fails to give a smooth dissection of the deep stroma to allow a clean interface and uniform bed for PD-DALK.

The Jacob modification of PD-DALK can be used as an immediate primary management technique for acute hydrops to prevent healing by scarring that can occur following conventional management strategies as described in their report.[6,7] It provides earlier and faster visual rehabilitation through a single-step surgery and decreases contact lens dependence. Patients are able to tolerate spectacles better after surgery as this single-staged treatment of acute hydrops gives visual, optical, topographic, biomechanical, and structural improvement in these already advanced cases of keratoconus. At the same time this technique avoids healing with scarring as is seen after conventional management of acute hydrops. Scar formation after conventional management strategies for acute hydrops can lead to difficult PD-DALK even if scar is in the periphery and, in case of scarring over the visual axis, can lead to the need for a PK with its attendant increased risk of graft rejection.

Discussion

Visual Recovery After DALK

Visual recovery is influenced, among other optical variables, by the transparency of corneal tissue. There is a concern that leaving behind residual stroma may cause interface haze or affect the visual outcome negatively due to abnormal light scattering of this layer. Fontana et al[1] found comparable visual function between DALK and PK when the recipient stroma is fully excised, and the DM is exposed, whereas visual results were inferior to those of PK when layers of stroma were left adherent to the DM, with creation of a stroma-stroma interface. They showed that manual stromal dissection, carried out in the very deep recipient stroma, results in the formation of an interface of poorer optical quality, leading to inferior visual results when compared with PK.[1] In one study, it was shown that when residual pre-Descemetic stroma was less than 20 μm, the results are comparable to PK, but where the stroma left is more than 80 μm, the visual acuity achieved can be inferior.[17]

There is a wide variation between studies comparing D-DALK and PD-DALK, which may be attributable to different indications for which DALK was attempted and differences in surgical techniques used, constantly evolving techniques over the study period and varying stromal bed left in various studies.[1] Sugita and Kondo[3], in 1997, reported no statistically significant difference in the visual acuity at 12 months after DALK among 80 eyes that had DM exposure and 40 eyes that had a fine layer of the deepest stroma left intraoperatively. Sarnicola et al,[10] in a retrospective study published in 2010, reported no difference in visual acuity between the PD-DALK and D-DALK groups at an average follow-up of 30.4 months, although the eyes in the D-DALK group seemed to have faster visual recovery. When comparing Anwar's technique and Melles' technique of DALK, it was found that imprecise judgment of corneal depth in the Melles' technique can prevent baring of DM and this may reduce the contrast sensitivity. However, the postoperative vision, refraction, aberration profile, and biomechanical strength of both techniques are comparable.[4] Acar et al[18] found similar outcomes over 12-month follow up in visual results of DALK eyes, though a delayed recovery was noted when big bubble was not achieved during surgery.

Studies Comparing D-DALK, PD-DALK, and PK Using In Vivo Confocal Microscopy

At 1 month after PD-DALK technique, the interface is characterized by a discontinuity in stromal extracellular architecture, with nonhomogeneous increased reflectivity due to tissue edema and presence of activated keratocytes located in the stromal layers adjacent to the interface optical section. The presence of activated keratocytes and tissue edema showed reduction at 6 months, and this may represent an index of tissue remodeling responsible for the observed decrease of reflectivity. The interface haze evaluated at the slit lamp, and the interface reflectivity seen on in vivo confocal microscopy post–PD-DALK, progressively decline over time and do not compromise the visual acuity eventually at 6 months. In the pre-Descemetic eyes, from 1 week after surgery, an increase in brightness of the interface when compared to D-DALK, due to presence of activated keratocytes, is detected by confocal microscopy. At around 10 to 12 weeks, the keratocyte morphology and reflectivity is shown to return to normal PD-DALK. This healing change is seen earlier in D-DALK eyes (4 to 6 weeks).[19]

The comparative study of in vivo confocal microscopy of the donor recipient interface in PD-DALK and D-DALK at 1 month showed that the peak of reflectivity at the interface after PD-DALK was significantly greater than the peak of reflectivity after D-DALK; however, at 6 months, the peak of reflectivity reduced to similar levels as the D-DALK eyes.[19]

Residual Bed Thickness

In PD-DALK cases, a wide variation of residual bed thickness (75 to 230 μm, average, 122±58 μm) was noted in a study by Schiano-Lomoriello et al.[20] They found that the reflectivity at donor recipient interface on confocal microscopy, though, was higher in the PD-DALK group, reduced to similar levels as in D-DALK group over a 6-month period.

Corneal Astigmatism

With regards to postoperative corneal astigmatism, topographically there was no difference found between D-DALK and PD-DALK.[17,20] Huang et al[21] found that in keratoconus, PD-DALK resulted in a slightly higher myopic refractive sphere postoperatively than D-DALK. Comparatively, the eye undergoing PK resulted in a lower myopia.

Quality of Vision

Pelli-Robson contrast sensitivity (PRCS), low-contrast visual acuity (LCVA) measurements, and effects of glare (ie, disability glare showed comparable LCVA and PRCS after PK and D-DALK), whereas both LCVA and PRCS were inferior after PD-DALK when compared with those after D-DALK. Subgroup analysis of DALK patients showed significantly better LCVA, with and without glare, in patients with DM exposure than in patients who underwent intrastromal manual dissection.[1] Fontana et al[1] noted that the presence of opacities in the interface, as seen on slit lamp, was recorded in a higher number of eyes after PD-DALK (40%) as compared to D-DALK (7%). Objective measurements of patients' optical characteristics show that total and higher-order aberrations are comparable after PK and DALK, despite 25% of DALK eyes presenting with some degree of interface opacities. This suggests that graft interface in DALK does not induce significant additional aberrations, measurable with the diagnostic instruments employed in the study.[1]

Conclusion

Where possible, D-DALK should be the goal; however, PD-DALK is a viable option where D-DALK is not possible, in order to prevent full-thickness transplant, which may subject the eye to possible risk of endothelial rejection. Though the final vision is achieved much later in PD-DALK, there is no significant compromise in final visual results. With the use of various dissection techniques, especially the groove and peel technique, it is possible to achieve an anterior lamellar surgery in difficult cases too, with results comparable to D-DALK.

References

1. Fontana L, Parente G, Sincich A, Tassinari G. Influence of graft-host interface on the quality of vision after deep anterior lamellar keratoplasty in patients with keratoconus. *Cornea.* 2011;30(5):497-502.
2. Shimazaki J. The evolution of lamellar keratoplasty. *Curr Opin Ophthalmol.* 2000;11(4):217-223.
3. Sugita J, Kondo J. Deep lamellar keratoplasty with complete removal of pathological stroma for vision improvement. *Br J Ophthalmol.* 1997;81(3):184-188.
4. Baradaran-Rafii A, Eslani M, Sadoughi M-M, Esfandiari H, Karimian F. Anwar versus Melles deep anterior lamellar keratoplasty for keratoconus: a prospective randomized clinical trial. *Ophthalmology.* 2013;120(2):252-259.
5. Mehta P, Rathi VM, Murthy SI. Deep anterior lamellar keratoplasty for the management of iatrogenic keratectasia occurring after hexagonal keratotomy. *Indian J Ophthalmol.* 2012;60(2):139-141.
6. Jacob S, Narasimhan S, Agarwal A, Sambath J, Umamaheshwari G, Saijimol AI. Primary modified predescemetic deep anterior lamellar keratoplasty in acute corneal hydrops. *Cornea.* 2018; 37(10):1328-1333.
7. Jacob S. Primary predescemetic DALK for acute hydrops Soosan Jacob with audio [video]. YouTube. https://www.youtube.com/watch?v=5ZeAXOmVDJw. Published June 14, 2018. Accessed September 27, 2018.
8. Jhanji V, Sharma N, Vajpayee RB. *Deep Anterior Lamellar Keratoplasty: Different Strokes.* New Delhi, India: Jaypee Brothers; 2012.
9. Anwar M, Teichmann KD. Big-bubble technique to bare Descemet's membrane in anterior lamellar keratoplasty. *J Cataract Refract Surg.* 2002;28(3):398-403.
10. Sarnicola V, Toro P, Gentile D, Hannush SB. Descemetic DALK and predescemetic DALK: outcomes in 236 cases of keratoconus. *Cornea.* 2010;29(1):53-59.
11. Marchini G, Mastropasqua L, Pedrotti E, Nubile M, Ciancaglini M, Sbabo A. Deep lamellar keratoplasty by intracorneal dissection: a prospective clinical and confocal microscopic study. *Ophthalmology.* 2006;113(8):1289-1300.
12. Swarup R, Bansal AG, Sangwan VS. No bubble, no trouble: the Groove & Peel Technique, a simplified approach to deep anterior lamellar keratoplasty. American Academy of Ophthalmology. https://www.aao.org/annual-meeting-video/no-bubble-trouble-groove--peel-technique-simplifie. Published December 1, 2008. Accessed February 18, 2019.
13. Chaniyara MH, Bafna R, Urkude J, Sharma N. Rescuing the host Descemet's membrane in full-thickness traumatic wound dehiscence in deep anterior lamellar keratoplasty: intraoperative optical coherence tomography (iOCT)-guided technique. *BMJ Case Rep.* 2017;2017:2017-221495. doi: 10.1136/bcr-2017-221495
14. Steven P, Le Blanc C, Lankenau E, et al. Optimising deep anterior lamellar keratoplasty (DALK) using intraoperative online optical coherence tomography (iOCT). *Br J Ophthalmol.* 2014;98(7):900-904.
15. De Benito-Llopis L, Mehta JS, Angunawela RI, Ang M, Tan DTH. Intraoperative anterior segment optical coherence tomography: a novel assessment tool during deep anterior lamellar keratoplasty. *Am J Ophthalmol.* 2014;157(2):334-341.

16. Lu Y, Grisolia ABD, Ge Y-R, et al. Comparison of femtosecond laser-assisted Descemetic and predescemetic lamellar keratoplasty for keratoconus. *Indian J Ophthalmol.* 2017;65(1):19-23.
17. Ardjomand N, Hau S, McAlister JC, et al. Quality of vision and graft thickness in deep anterior lamellar and penetrating corneal allografts. *Am J Ophthalmol.* 2007;143(2):228-235.
18. Acar BT, Vural ET, Acar S. Is it really important to form a big bubble in DALK to enhance the visual acuity? *Eye Contact Lens.* 2012;38(5):274-277.
19. Abdelkader A, Kaufman HE. Descemetic versus pre-Descemetic lamellar keratoplasty: clinical and confocal study. *Cornea.* 2011;30(11):1244-1252.
20. Schiano-Lomoriello D, Colabelli-Gisoldi RA, Nubile M, et al. Descemetic and predescemetic DALK in keratoconus patients: a clinical and confocal perspective study. *BioMed Res Int.* 2014;2014:123156.
21. Huang T, Hu Y, Gui M, Hou C, Zhang H. Comparison of refractive outcomes in three corneal transplantation techniques for keratoconus. *Graefes Arch Clin Exp Ophthalmol.* 2015;253(11):1947-1953.

Please see videos on the accompanying website at
www.healio.com/books/DALKvideos

7

The Melles Technique

C. Maya Tong, BSc, MD; Jack Parker, MD, PhD;
Korine van Dijk, BOptom, PhD; Rénuka S. Birbal, MD;
and Gerrit R. J. Melles, MD, PhD

Deep anterior lamellar keratoplasty (DALK) is designed to exchange healthy donor corneal stroma for recipient pathologic corneal stroma. Unlike its predecessor, penetrating keratoplasty (PK), DALK leaves the recipient Descemet's membrane (DM) and endothelium intact. Broadly speaking, there are 2 basic, competing, surgical strategies for DALK: those relying on injection and those relying on manual dissection. Melles Manual DALK (MM-DALK) falls into the latter category; it is unique in that, unlike other manual techniques, MM-DALK facilitates precise, reliable dissection down to the level of the DM by use of a phenomenon known as the *air-endothelial reflex*.[1,2]

Background

Anterior lamellar keratoplasty (ALK) was first developed over 150 years ago.[3] Early attempts at the operation, where the recipient cornea was dissected near the DM, were made as early as the 1950s by Hallermann.[4] While structurally and technically successful, these early efforts were largely regarded, both optically and functionally, as failures, because the visual results of the early anterior lamellar transplants were often far inferior to those achieved by penetrating grafts.[5] The explanation for this underperformance was that total removal of the recipient stroma, down to the DM, was difficult to achieve by the usual means of manual dissection from the corneal surface. The layers of stroma inevitably left behind would interact negatively with

Jacob S, ed. *Mastering DALK: A Video Textbook on Deep Anterior Lamellar Keratoplasty* (pp 81-92).

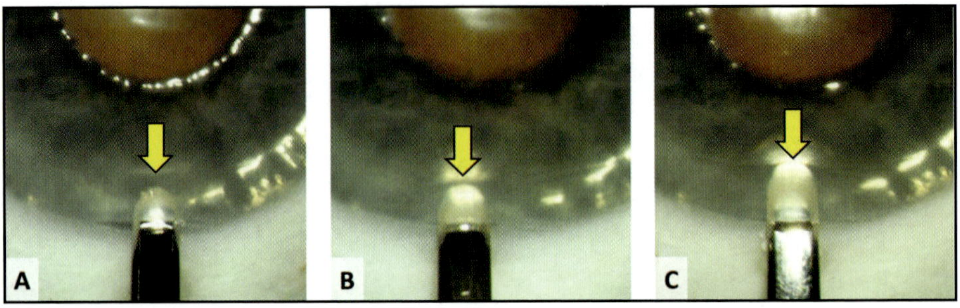

Figure 7-1. Surgical views demonstrating the determination of the dissection depth in a human donor eye. The anterior chamber has been filled with air. (A) In between the blade tip and the air-to-endothelial interface light reflex, a dark band (arrow) is visible. (B) The dark band decreases in width when the blade is advanced into the deeper stromal layers because it reflects unincised posterior corneal tissue. (C) When the blade appears to touch the air-to-endothelial interface, a stromal dissection level just anterior to the posterior corneal surface is reached.

the donor tissue, producing haze at the graft interface and spoiling the transplant's optical performance.[6] Therefore, major attempts at ALK were largely abandoned for decades until new methods for more complete recipient stromal removal could be discovered.

Important technical improvements were made in the early 1990s, when Amayem and Anwar [7] published that injection of saline into the deep corneal stroma could often result in a cleavage plane just above the DM. Several years later, Anwar and Teichmann[8] refined the technique utilizing air instead of saline, effectively developing the big bubble strategy for DALK. Around the same time, it was also independently discovered that deep injections of viscoelastic could yield similar results.[9] Nevertheless, a major problem with these injection techniques was their reliability; big bubbles were not always achieved, and, even worse, approximately 10% to 50% of attempts resulted in inadvertent DM perforation secondary to rapid expansion of the injected material.[9-16] This unpredictability in outcome drove the search for a new technique that would permit a controlled separation of the recipient stroma from its DM, and gave rise to the development of the MM-DALK method.

The Melles Manual DALK Surgical Technique

The MM-DALK operation is based on a single observation and relies on a specialized set of instruments. The observation is this: if the recipient anterior chamber is completely filled with air, when instruments are inserted into the peripheral cornea, a reflection of the tip of those instruments appears. The deeper the instrument is pressed into the cornea, the closer the reflection appears to the instrument, such that, when the 2 are nearly touching, a stromal dissection level just anterior to the posterior corneal surface has been achieved (Figure 7-1). This air-endothelial reflex provides an immediate, ever-present indication of the depth of the ongoing dissection and thereby enables a controlled, precise manual separation of the host stroma away from the underlying DM.[1,2] After a superior peritomy is performed and a 5-mm corneoscleral tunnel is fashioned using a crescent blade, the anterior chamber is filled with air (Figure 7-2). A specialized set of 3 spatulas (Melles spatula set; DORC International BV) is then employed. These spatulas have red, white, and blue handles corresponding to their increasing lengths and curvatures. They are used in sequence to bluntly dissect through the recipient cornea, from limbus-to-limbus, 360° around, guided by the air-endothelial reflex (see Figure 7-2).[1,2]

After this stromal dissection is completed, the air is removed from the anterior chamber and viscoelastic is injected into the dissected stromal pocket. The anterior corneal surface is trephined away and the donor lamellar graft is sutured into position (see Figure 7-2).[1,2]

Preoperative Considerations and Surgical Indications

The most common indications for MM-DALK are advanced keratoconus, or a patient with a history of corneal hydrops treated conventionally, which is typically regarded as a contraindication to big bubble DALK due to an increased risk of DM perforation.[17-21] The Jacob modification of pre-Descemetic DALK has been described for primary management of acute hydrops to prevent the scarring that is generally seen following conventional management.[22,23] Faster visual rehabilitation through a single staged surgery and decreased contact lens dependence are other advantages, as are visual, optical, topographic, biomechanical, and structural improvement in these advanced cases of keratoconus.

Other less common indications include post-herpetic/traumatic corneal scarring and a variety of corneal stromal dystrophies.[24-26] Unquestionably, the health of the corneal endothelium is a main criterion for deciding if a DALK procedure is indicated. The best surgical candidates are adults with 2 severely visually impaired eyes, because psychological surveys have demonstrated that patient satisfaction with corneal replacement for keratoconus depends more on the operated eye becoming the better seeing eye, rather than the absolute level of visual improvement the surgery yields.[27-29] Few studies of pediatric DALK (of any technique) have been conducted, but patient ability and willingness to cooperate are generally correlated with operative success.[30,31]

MM-DALK may be regarded as a minimally invasive procedure, because nearly all its steps are extraocular, and do not involve manipulations within the globe.[1,2] As a result, MM-DALK may be performed with only retrobulbar anesthesia. Obtaining a soft eye may be the single most important pre-surgical step, as the manual stromal dissection is made substantially more difficult by significant posterior pressure, which raises the chances of inadvertent DM perforation.[2,26] Therefore, an effective retrobulbar block, followed by digital ocular massage and a Honan balloon, are strongly advised. Intraoperatively, the patient should be placed in a proper anti-Trendelenberg position, and careful attention should be paid to the tightness of the speculum to ensure that excessive pressure is not being applied to the globe.

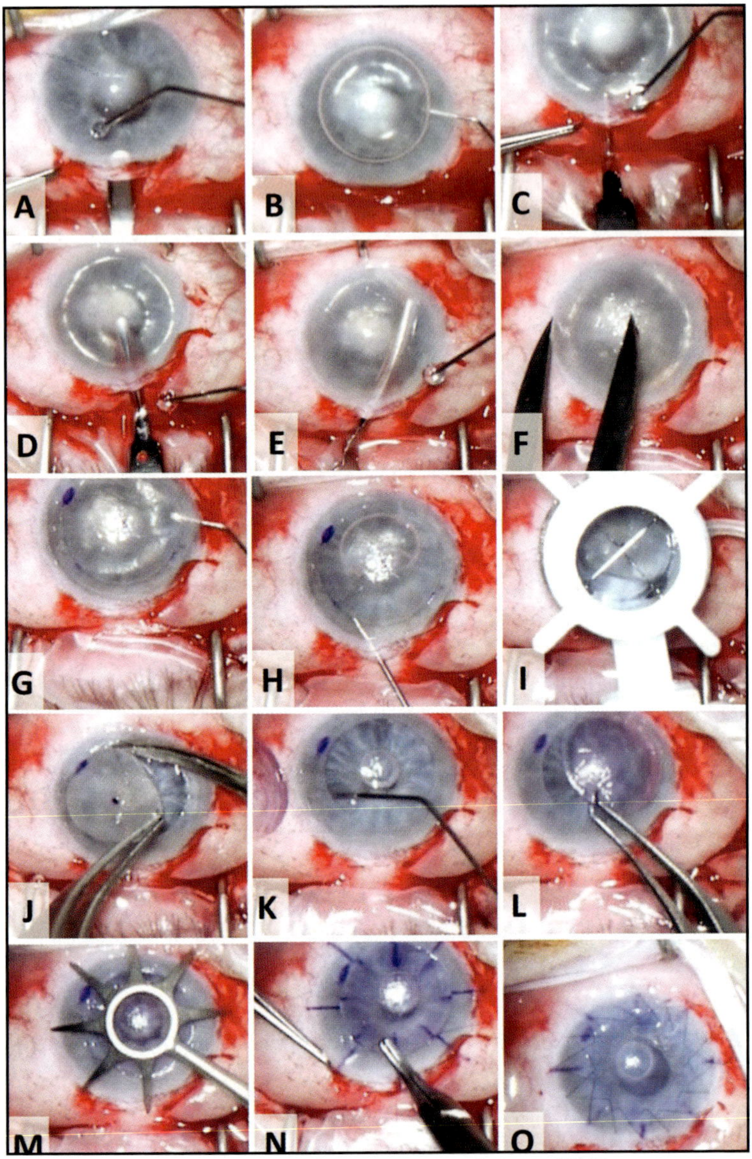

Figure 7-2. Surgical stills demonstrating the MM-DALK technique. (A) After a superior peritomy is performed and a 5-mm corneoscleral tunnel is fashioned using a crescent blade, (B) the anterior chamber is filled with air through a side port. Then, (C-E) a deep stromal dissection up to the limbus over 360° is completed with 3 increasing sizes spatulas. The thin black line alongside the spatula serves as an indication for dissection depth. (F) After marking the center of the cornea and (G) removing most air from the anterior chamber, (H) the dissected pocket is filled with viscoelastic to separate the DM from the posterior stroma. Next, (I) with a Hessburg-Barron trephine the anterior corneal lamella is trephined until the viscoelastic escapes (J) and excised while leaving the DM in situ. (K) Note the smooth recipient bed, which is rinsed with balanced salt solution (L) before an anterior lamellar donor button is placed onto the recipient bed. Finally, (M, N) the donor and recipient corneal surfaces are marked with an 8-incision radial keratotomy marker, (O) and the donor button is sutured in place with 2 running sutures.

Post-Surgical Results

The visual results of MM-DALK likely depend on whether deep stromal dissection is successfully achieved, but, given that, may equal those achieved by big bubble DALK and conventional PK, with an average resultant best spectacle-corrected visual acuity of 20/40 (0.5).[32-39] The endothelial cell density of MM-DALK–operated eyes tends to be higher than that found with big bubble DALK, suggesting that rapid bubble expansion may be somehow traumatic to the recipient corneal endothelium.[40,41]

Compared to PK, DALK generally results in more postoperative myopia, because the resultant corneas are often steeper by, on average, 2 diopters (D); this may be because DALK avoids the intraoperative collapse of the anterior chamber and angle that is entailed by PK.[42-44] The degree of myopia may, however, be decreased by using same size grafts. Whereas, after PK, approximately 10% of operated eyes may require rigid contact lens fitting to achieve satisfactory visual results, no such figures have been published for big bubble or MM-DALK.[45-50]

Theoretically, DALK may permit earlier suture removal compared to PK and, therefore, more rapid visual stability. This claim has been occasionally extended to argue that DALK performed with the assistance of the femtosecond laser for shaping the edges of the donor and recipient tissues into interlocking configurations may be conducive to even greater stability and earlier suture removal compared to big bubble and MM-DALK.[51-53] However, the only study on the subject to specifically examine the issue failed to corroborate this hypothesis.[54] Another limitation of the femtosecond laser for DALK is that the device has demonstrated a surprising inability to perform adequately deep dissections in the recipient cornea. Specifically, deep laser cutting depths have been shown to generate ridges in the bed of the recipient cornea, and these ridges may undermine the optical performance of the eye compared to the dissections produced by big bubble and MM-DALK methods.[55,56]

One criticism of both PK and DALK is that neither operation tends to prevent disease recurrence; that is, resumed corneal ectasia in the transplanted tissue or at the graft-host junction.[57-65] Infiltration of the donor tissue with pathologic recipient keratocytes is one proposed mechanism for such recurrences.[66] If this is correct, then DALK may actually carry a somewhat higher risk than PK, as more of the recipient cornea is left in-situ, unexcised, in proportion to the depth and diameter of the achieved dissection.

Surgical and Post-Surgical Complications

DALK's most common complication is intraoperative DM perforation, which may occur in approximately 10% of eyes operated with both the MM- and big bubble DALK techniques.[8,9,11,12,37,67] In the latter, perforation may frequently necessitate conversion to PK because large surface incisions into the recipient cornea have already been created; the intrastromal air injection is usually performed after partial-thickness surface trephination.[68,69] In contrast, with MM-DALK, perforation may be managed expectantly by aborting the operation and permitting the cornea to heal, thereby enabling another attempt at DALK in the future.

Another commonly discussed complication after DALK is graft failure; this remains a highly controversial topic today, mostly secondary to disputes over terminology. Specifically, graft failure originally referred to corneal decompensation stemming from donor endothelial cell death or depletion.[70] This type of graft failure is exceedingly rare with DALK. The average life expectancy of an anterior lamellar transplant following uncomplicated surgery has been estimated at approximately 50 years, compared to approximately 18 years following PK.[71] However, it has recently also become popular to use the term graft failure to describe an optically undesirable result following otherwise successful DALK surgery. These underperforming grafts may, for example, feature dense interface haze that limits the visual performance of the eye that received the transplant.[72] Some studies have decided to classify these optically disappointing DALKs as *failed grafts*; however, it should be noted that graft failure in this sense is not the same as it has been conventionally understood. Moreover, it means special caution must be applied when comparing the rates or incidences of graft failure between PK and DALK, as different outcomes may be lumped under the same broad term. Therefore, it may be advisable to distinguish between cellular and optical graft failure, and to distinguish clearly what is meant in each instance.[73]

No comparative studies yet exist between MM-DALK and big bubble DALK for allograft reaction or cellular graft failure. However, as cell densities tend to be higher after mm- compared to big bubble DALK, and the occurrences of inadvertent DM perforation may tend to be lower, graft survival may be longer in the manual method.[38,39,69]

Melles Manual DALK Alternative and the Future of Anterior Lamellar Keratoplasty

Although DALK confers a number of advantages over conventional PK for many patients, significant, intrinsic drawbacks to the operation nevertheless remain. These include the necessity to make large surface incisions in the recipient cornea, the requirement for long-standing corneal sutures, the use of cellular donor material, the ongoing risk for allograft reaction and graft rejection, and the demand for significant extended follow-up examinations.[74-77] All of these postoperative risks and obligations are entailed by the inherent nature of DALK itself, and, therefore, are not likely to be resolved by any future advances in operative technique, instrumentation, or medication. If they are to be definitively solved or avoided, some entirely new surgical technique may be necessary.

It has been recently shown that alternative techniques, such as UV–cross-linking (UV-CXL), may be changing the role of DALK for anterior corneal diseases. The introduction of UV-CXL in Europe effectively slowed or halted the progression of keratoconus, and may have contributed to a 25% decrease in DALKs being performed in the years following its nationwide.[78,79] The frequency of DALK in the United States, on the other hand, remained stable over the last 10 years.[80] However, with

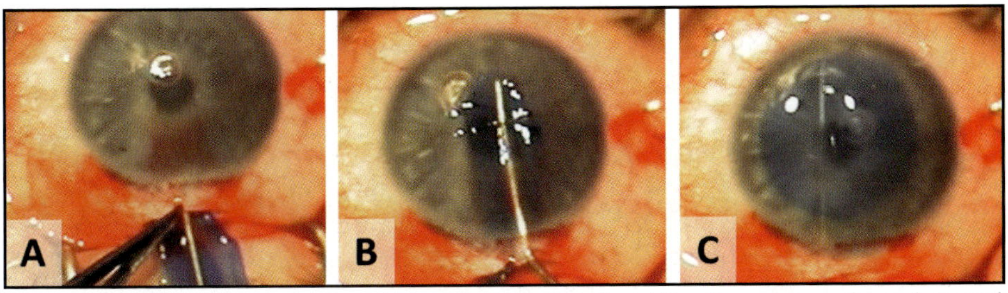

Figure 7-3. Surgical views of an eye during BL transplantation. After the creation of a mid-stromal pocket using the MM-DALK dissection technique, (A) a stained BL graft is inserted into the pocket through a glide and (B) carefully unfolded and centered with a 30-gauge air cannula. (C) At the end of the surgery, the BL graft is sandwiched between the anterior and posterior stromal layers. No sutures are required to fixate the graft or to close the tunnel incision.

the approval of UV-CXL by the US Food and Drug Administration in April 2016 for treatment of patients with progressive keratoconus and post-LASIK ectasia, the United States may also experience a decrease in frequency of DALK in the coming years.

In addition to the evolving role of UV-CXL, a new operation has been described as an alternative to PK and DALK for patients with advanced keratoconus: Bowman layer (BL) transplantation. The purpose of the operation is to arrest and, to some extent, reverse the progression of disease in patients who are not candidates for either UV-CXL or intrastromal corneal ring segments.[21,81]

The BL surgery is performed by making a manual, mid-stromal dissection within the recipient keratoconic cornea using the standard MM-DALK dissection spatulas. An isolated BL graft is inserted and unfolded within this created corneal pocket at a depth of approximately 50% (Figure 7-3).[21,81] The major advantages of BL transplantation include halting corneal ectasia in approximately 90% of transplanted eyes, stabilizing and flattening the cornea by about 8 D after surgery, and decreasing risk for allograft and graft rejection, while suture related complications cannot occur (Figures 7-4 and 7-5). Further, the operation can be considered reversible in that, if the desired outcome is not obtained, a DALK or PK can always be performed at a later date.[21,81,82] BL transplantation may therefore confer many of the same advantages as UV-CXL and intrastromal corneal ring segments, but for patients whose corneas are too thin or steep to qualify for either of these operations.[21,81,82]

Conclusion

The primary reason for preferring MM-DALK over big bubble DALK and other manual techniques may be the unequaled level of visualization and control that the technique offers compared to its competitors. The tactic may therefore be regarded as more repeatable and perhaps safer. Its disadvantages, however, include that the technique is skill-dependent and relies on meticulous attention to detail, because the depth of dissection must be continuously monitored. Manual dissection may

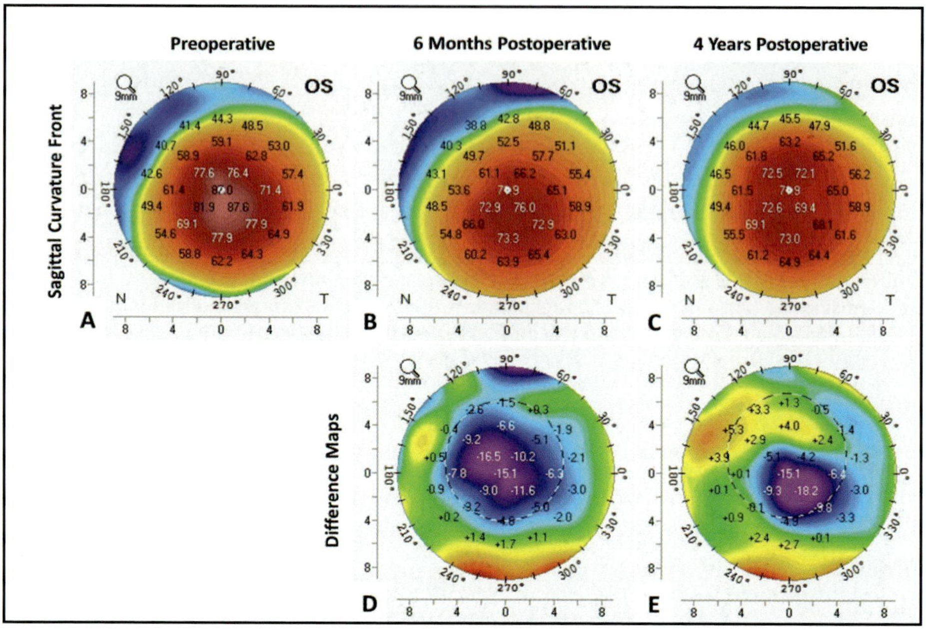

Figure 7-4. Topographic maps of a cornea (A) prior to, (B) 6 months, and (C) 4 years after BL transplantation. (D, E) Note the significant corneal flattening displayed in the difference maps from preoperative to 6 months and 4 years postoperatively. (N = nasal; T = temporal.)

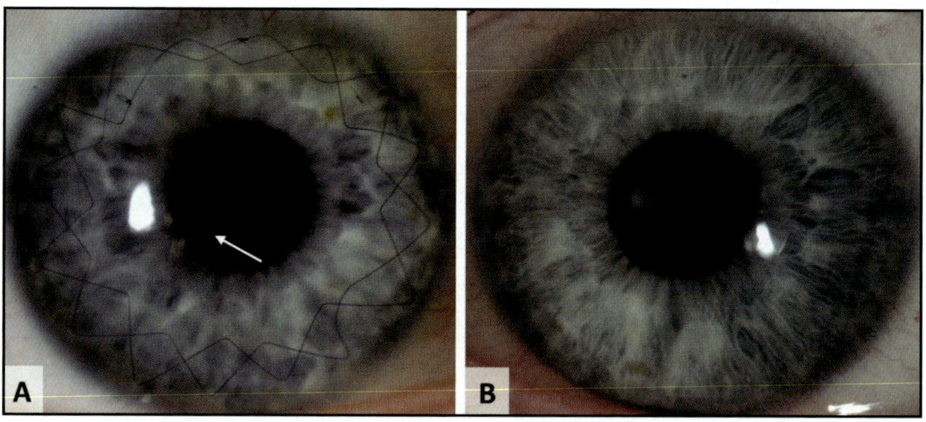

Figure 7-5. Slit lamp images of a patient who underwent (A) MM-DALK in the right eye and (B) BL transplantation in the left eye; both images were obtained 6 months postoperatively. (A) Note the wrinkling of the DM (white arrow head) in the right eye. (B) The left cornea is clear, without interface haze or stromal reaction.

also be more time consuming compared to big bubble DALK. The operation also demands a specialized set of instruments that must be specially ordered. The biggest problem with the surgery, however, is that it fails to resolve DALK's most significant postoperative) drawbacks, which are related to the surface incisions, sutures, and cellular donor material. No DALK technique of any sort adequately addresses these significant challenges, and, therefore, some fundamentally new operation may be appropriate. These are the motivations that inspired a less interventionist, more specific alternative for patients with advanced keratoconus; namely, BL transplantation. BL transplantation is still a relatively new operation, and its first patients are now only 8 years removed from surgery. Nevertheless, depending on the results of further studies, this operation may be poised to displace nearly full-thickness corneal replacement for patients with advanced keratoconus, much as the endothelial keratoplasty techniques displaced PK for patients with Fuchs' dystrophy.

References

1. Melles GR, Rietveld FJ, Beekhuis WH, Binder PS. A technique to visualize corneal incision and lamellar dissection depth during surgery. *Cornea*. 1999;19:80-86.
2. Melles GRJ, Lander F, Rietveld FJR, Beekhuis WH, Binder PS. A new surgical technique for deep stromal, anterior lamellar keratoplasty. *Br J Ophthalmol*. 1999;83:327-333.
3. Mühlbauer FX. Ueber transplantation der cornea; Gekrönte Preisschrift. München, Jos. Lindauer, 1840. (Abstract) In: Schmidt CC, ed. *Jahrbücher der in und Ausländischen Gesamten Medizin*. Leipzig, Germany: Otto Wigand; 1842:267-268.
4. Hallermann W. Verschiedenes über Keratoplastik. *Klin Monatsbl Augenheilkd*. 1959;135:252-259.
5. Morrison JC, Swan KC. Full-thickness lamellar keratoplasty. A histologic study in human eyes. *Ophthalmology*. 1982;89:715-719.
6. Krachmer JH, Mannis MJ, Holland EJ. *Cornea: Fundamentals, Diagnosis, and Management*. St. Louis, MO: Mosby Elsevier; 2011.
7. Amayem AF, Anwar M. Fluid lamellar keratoplasty in keratoconus. *Ophthalmology*. 2000;107:76-79.
8. Anwar M, Teichmann KD. Big-bubble technique to bare Descemet's membrane in anterior lamellar keratoplasty. *J Cataract Refract Surg*. 2002;28:398-403.
9. Melles GR, Remeijer L, Geerards AJ, Beekhuis WH. A quick surgical technique for deep anterior lamellar keratoplasty using visco-dissection. *Cornea*. 2000;19:427-432.
10. Den S, Shimmura S, Tsubota K, Shimazaki J. Impact of the Descemet membrane perforation on surgical outcomes after deep lamellar keratoplasty. *Am J Ophthalmol*. 2007;143:750-754.
11. Feizi S, Javadi MA, Jamali H, Mirbabaee F. Deep anterior lamellar keratoplasty in patients with keratoconus: big-bubble technique. *Cornea*. 2010;29:177-182.
12. Leccisotti A. Descemet's membrane perforation during deep anterior lamellar keratoplasty: prognosis. *J Cataract Refract Surg*. 2007;33:825-829.
13. Goweida MB. Intraoperative review of different bubble types formed during pneumodissection (big-bubble) deep anterior lamellar keratoplasty. *Cornea*. 2015;34:621-624.
14. Michieletto P, Balestrazzi A, Balestrazzi A, Mazzotta C, Occhipinti I, Rossi T. Factors predicting unsuccessful big bubble deep lamellar anterior keratoplasty. *Ophthalmologica*. 2006;220:379-382.
15. Feizi S, Faramarzi A, Javadi MA, Jafarinasab MR. Modified big-bubble deep anterior lamellar keratoplasty using peripheral air injection. *Br J Ophthalmol*. 2014;98:1597-1600.
16. Feizi S, Daryabari SH, Najdi D, Javadi MA, Farimian F. Big-bubble deep anterior lamellar keratoplasty using central vs peripheral air injection: a clinical trial. *Eur J Ophthalmol*. 2016;26:297-302.

17. Anwar M. Planned near Descemet's membrane dissection using air and fluid. In: John T, ed. *Surgical Techniques in Anterior and Posterior Lamellar Corneal Surgery.* New Delhi, India: Jaypee Brothers; 2006:126-133.
18. Fogla R. Deep anterior lamellar keratoplasty in the management of keratoconus. *Indian J Ophthalmol.* 2013;61:465-468.
19. Parker JS, van Dijk K, Melles GR. Treatment options for advanced keratoconus: a review. *Surv Ophthalmol.* 2015;60:459-480.
20. Fan Gaskin JC, Patel DV, McGhee CN. Acute corneal hydrops in keratoconus—new perspectives. *Am J Ophthalmol.* 2014;157:921-928.
21. Jabbarvand M, Mohammadpour M. Deep lamellar keratoplasty in keratoconus with healed hydrops. *Cornea.* 2008;27:1100.
22. Jacob S, Narasimhan S, Agarwal A, Sambath J, Umamaheshwari G, Saijimol AI. Primary modified predescemetic deep anterior lamellar keratoplasty in acute corneal hydrops. *Cornea.* 2018;37(10):1328-1333.
23. Jacob S. Primary predescemetic DALK for acute hydrops Soosan Jacob with audio [video]. YouTube. https://www.youtube.com/watch?v=5ZeAXOmVDJw. Published June 14, 2018. Accessed September 27, 2018.
24. Millar MJ, Maloof A. Deep lamellar keratoplasty for pellucid marginal degeneration review of management options for corneal perforation. *Cornea.* 2008;27:953-956.
25. Kawashima M, Kawakita T, Den S, Shimmura S, Tsubota K, Shimazaki J. Comparison of deep lamellar keratoplasty and penetrating keratoplasty for lattice and macular corneal dystrophies. *Am J Ophthalmol.* 2006;142:304-309.
26. Karimian F, Feizi S. Deep anterior lamellar keratoplasty: indications, surgical techniques, and complications. *Middle East Afr J Ophthalmol.* 2010;17:28-37.
27. Mendes F, Schaumberg DA, Navon S, Steinert R, Sugar J, Holland EJ, Dana MR. Assessment of visual function after corneal transplantation: the quality of life and psychometric assessment after corneal transplantation (Q-PACT) study. *Am J Ophthalmol.* 2003;135:785-793.
28. Uiters E, van den Borne B, van der Horst FG, Völker-Dieben HJ. Patient satisfaction after corneal transplantation. *Cornea.* 2001;20:687-694.
29. Williams KA, Ash JK, Pararajasegaram P, Dipl H, Coster DJ. Long-term outcome after corneal transplantation: visual result and patient perception of success. *Ophthalmology.* 1991;98:651-657.
30. Singh D, Vanathi M, Gupta C, Gupta N, Tandon R. Outcomes of deep anterior lamellar keratoplasty following autologous simple limbal epithelial transplant in pediatric unilateral severe chemical injury. *Indian J Ophthalmol.* 2017;65:217-222.
31. Harding SA, Nischal KK, Upponi-Patil A, Fowler DJ. Indications and outcomes of deep anterior lamellar keratoplasty in children. *Ophthalmology.* 2010;117:2191-2195.
32. Fontana L, Parente G, Sincich A, Tassinari G. Influence of graft-host interface on the quality of vision after deep anterior lamellar keratoplasty in patients with keratoconus. *Cornea.* 2011;30:497-502.
33. Funnell CL, Ball J, Noble BA. Comparative cohort study of the outcomes of deep lamellar keratoplasty and penetrating keratoplasty for keratoconus. *Eye (Lond).* 2006;20:527-532.
34. Han DC, Mehta JS, Por YM, Htoon HM, Tan DT. Comparison of outcomes of lamellar keratoplasty and penetrating keratoplasty in keratoconus. *Am J Ophthalmol.* 2009;148:744-751.
35. Javadi MA, Motlagh BF, Jafarinasab MR, Rabbanikhah Z. Outcomes of penetrating keratoplasty in keratoconus. *Cornea.* 2005;24:941-946.
36. Jones MN, Armitage WJ, Ayliffe W, Larkin DF, Kaye SB; NHSBT Ocular Tissue Advisory Group and Contributing Ophthalmologists (OTAG Audit Study 5). Penetrating and deep anterior lamellar keratoplasty for keratoconus: a comparison of graft outcomes in the United Kingdom. *Invest Ophhthalmol Vis Sci.* 2009;50:5625-5629.
37. Kim MH, Chung TY, Chung ES. A retrospective contralateral study comparing deep anterior lamellar keratoplasty with penetrating keratoplasty. *Cornea.* 2013;32:385-389.
38. Smadja D, Colin J, Kreuger RR. Outcomes of deep anterior lamellar keratoplasty for keratoconus: learning curve and advantages of the big bubble technique. *Cornea.* 2012;31:859-863.

39. Keane M, Coster D, Ziaei M, Williams K. Deep anterior lamellar keratoplasty versus penetrating keratoplasty for treating keratoconus. *Cochrane Database Syst Rev.* 2014;22:CD009700.
40. Borderie VM, Werthel AL, Touzeau O, Allouch C, Boutboul S, Laroche L. Comparison of techniques used for removing the recipient stroma in anterior lamellar keratoplasty. *Arch Ophthalmol.* 2008;126:31-37.
41. Cheng YY, Visser N, Schouten JS, et al. Endothelial cell loss and visual outcome of deep anterior lamellar keratoplasty versus penetrating keratoplasty: a randomized multicenter clinical trial. *Ophthalmology.* 2011;188:302-309.
42. Amayem AF, Hamdi IM, Hamdi MM. Refractive and visual outcomes of penetrating keratoplasty versus keep anterior lamellar keratoplasty with hydrodissection for treatment of keratoconus. *Cornea.* 2013;32:e2-e5.
43. Borderie VM, Georgeon C, Borderie M, Bouheraoua N, Touzeau O, Laroche L. Corneal radius of curvature after anterior lamellar versus penetrating keratoplasty. *Graefes Arch Clin Exp Ophthalmol.* 2014;252:449-456.
44. Kim KH, Choi SH, Ahn K, Chung ES, Chung TY. Comparison of refractive changes after deep anterior lamellar keratoplasty and penetrating keratoplasty for keratoconus. *Jpn J Ophthalmol.* 2011;55:93-97.
45. Geerards AJ, Vreugdenhil W, Khazen A. Incidence of rigid gas-permeable contact lens wear after keratoplasty for keratoconus. *Eye Contact Lens.* 2006;32:207-210.
46. Lim L, Pesudovs K, Coster DJ. Penetrating keratoplasty for keratoconus: visual outcome and success. *Ophthalmology.* 2000;107:1125-1131.
47. Price FW Jr, Whitson WE, Marks RG. Progression of visual acuity after penetrating keratoplasty. *Ophthalmology.* 1991;98:1177-1185.
48. Severinsky B, Behrman S, Frucht-Pery J, Solomon A. Scleral contact lenses for visual rehabilitation after penetrating keratoplasty: long term outcomes. *Cont Lens Anterior Eye.* 2014;37:196-202.
49. Silbiger JS, Cohen EJ, Laibson PR. The rate of visual recovery after penetrating keratoplasty for keratoconus. *Cont Lens Anterior Eye.* 1996;22:266-269.
50. Sutton G, Hodge C, McGhee CN. Rapid visual recovery after penetrating keratoplasty for keratoconus. *Clin Experiment Ophthalmol.* 2008;36:725-730.
51. Lu Y, Yang L, Ge, Y, Chen X, Huang Z. Femtosecond laser-assisted anterior lamellar keratoplasty for the treatment of stromal corneal pathology. *BMC Ophthalmol.* 2015;15:15
52. Fung SS, Aiello F, Maurino V. Outcomes of femtosecond laser-assisted mushroom-configuration keratoplasty in advanced keratoconus. *Arch Ophthalmol.* 2012;130:776-782.
53. Chen Y, Hu DN, Xia Y, Yang L, Xue C, Huang Z. Comparison of femtosecond laser-assisted deep anterior lamellar keratoplasty and penetrating keratoplasty for keratoconus. *BMC Ophthalmol.* 2015;15:144.
54. Shehadeh-Mashor R, Chan CC, Bahar I, Lichtinger A, Yeung SN, Rootman DS. Comparison between femtosecond laser mushroom configuration and manual trephine straight-edge configuration deep anterior lamellar keratoplasty. *Br J Ophthalmol.* 2014;98:35-39.
55. Yokogawa H, Tang M, Li Y, Chamberlain W, Huang D. Deep laser-assisted lamellar anterior keratoplasty with microkeratome-cut grafts. *Cornea.* 2016;35:706-712.
56. Zhang C, Bald M, Tang M, Li Y, Huang D. Interface quality of different corneal lamellar-cut depths for femtosecond laser-assisted lamellar anterior keratoplasty. *J Cataract Refract Surg.* 2015;41:827-835.
57. Bechrakis N, Blom ML, Stark WJ, Green WR. Recurrent keratoconus. *Cornea.* 1994;13:73-77.
58. Dang TQ, Molchan RP, Taylor KR, Reilly CD, Panday VA, Caldwell MC. Novel approach for the treatment of corneal ectasia in a graft. *Cornea.* 2014;33:310-312.
59. Fukuoka S, Honda N, Ono K, Mimura T, Usui T, Amano S. Extended long-term results of penetrating keratoplasty for keratoconus. *Cornea.* 2010;29:528-530.
60. Hayes S, Young R, Boote C, Hawksworth N, Huang Y, Meek KM. A structural investigation of corneal graft failure in suspected recurrent keratoconus. *Eye (Lond).* 2010;24:728-734.
61. Lim L, Pesudovs K, Goggin M, Coster DJ. Late onset post-keratoplasty astigmatism in patients with keratoconus: indications and outcomes. *Br J Ophthalmol.* 2004;88:371-376.

62. Nirankari VS, Karesh J, Bastion F, Lakhanpal V, Billings E. Recurrence of keratoconus in donor cornea 22 years after successful keratoplasty. *Br J Ophthalmol.* 1983;67:23-28.
63. Niziol LM, Musch DC, Gillespie BW, Marcotte LM, Sugar A. Long-term outcomes in patients who received a corneal graft for keratoconus between 1980 and 1986. *Am J Ophthalmol.* 2013;155:213-219.
64. Patel SV, Malta JB, Banitt MR, et al. Recurrent ectasia in corneal grafts and outcomes of repeat keratoplasty for keratoconus. *Br J Ophthalmol.* 2009;93:191-197.
65. Yeniad B, Alparslan N, Akarcay K. Eye rubbing as an apparent cause of recurrent keratoconus. *Cornea.* 2009;28:477-479.
66. Bourges JL, Savoldelli M, Dighiero P, et al. Recurrence of keratoconus characteristics: a clinical and histological follow-up analysis of donor grafts. *Ophthalmology.* 2003;110:1920-1925.
67. Villarrubia A, Fuentes-Páez G, Dapena I, Palacín E. Deep anterior lamellar keratoplasty with Melles' technique: mid-term clinical outcome. *J Emmetropia.* 2010;1:182-186.
68. Anwar HM, El-Danasoury A, Hashem AN. The use of fibrin glue to seal Descemet membrane microperforations occurring during deep anterior lamellar keratoplasty. *Cornea.* 2012;31:1193-1196.
69. Sutiga J, Kondo J. Deep lamellar keratoplasty with complete removal of pathological stroma for vision improvement. *Br J Ophthalmol.* 1997;81:184-188.
70. Sharma N, Kandar AK, Singh Titiyal J. Stromal rejection after big bubble deep anterior lamellar keratoplasty: case series and review of literature. *Eye Contact Lens.* 2013;39:194-198.
71. Borderie VM, Sandali O, Bullet J. Long-term results of deep anterior lamellar versus penetrating keratoplasty. *Ophthalmology.* 2012;119:249-255.
72. Coster DJ, Lowe MT, Keane MC, Williams KA; Australian Corneal Graft Registry Contributors. A comparison of lamellar and penetrating keratoplasty outcomes: a registry study. *Ophthalmology.* 2014;121:979-987.
73. Baydoun L, Melles GR. Refining the terminology of graft failure in reports on endothelial keratoplasty outcomes. *JAMA Ophthalmol.* 2016;134:125-126.
74. Williams KA, Muehlberg SM, Lewis RF, Coster DJ. How successful is corneal transplantation? A report from the Australian Corneal Graft Register. *Eye (Lond).* 1995;9:219-227.
75. de Toledo JA, de la Paz MF, Barraquer RI, Barraquer J. Long-term progression of astigmatism after penetrating keratoplasty for keratoconus: evidence of late recurrence. *Cornea.* 2003;22:317-323.
76. Elder MJ, Stack RR. Globe rupture following penetrating keratoplasty: how often, why, and what can we do to prevent it? *Cornea.* 2004;23:776-780.
77. Nagra PK, Hammersmith KM, Rapuano CJ, Laibson PR, Cohen EJ. Wound dehiscence after penetrating keratoplasty. *Cornea.* 2006;25:132-135.
78. Godefrooij DA, Gans R, Imhof SM, Wisse RPL. Nationwide reduction in the number of corneal transplantations for keratoconus following the implementation of cross-linking. *Acta Ophthalmol.* 2016;94:675-678.
79. Sandvik GF, Thorsrud A, Raen M, Ostern AE, Saethre M, Drolsum L. Does corneal collagen cross-linking reduce the need for keratoplasties in patients with keratoconus? *Cornea.* 2015;34:991-995.
80. Park CYP, Lee JK, Gore PK, Lim C, Chuck RS. Keratoplasty in the United States: a 10-year review from 2005 through 2014. *Ophthalmology.* 2015;112:2432-2442.
81. van Dijk K, Parker J, Tong CM, Ham L, Lie JT, Groeneveld-van Beek EA, Melles, GRJ. Midstromal isolated Bowman layer graft for reduction of advanced keratoconus: a technique to postpone penetrating or deep anterior lamellar keratoplasty. *JAMA Ophthalmol.* 2014;132:495-501.
82. van Dijk K, Liarakos V, Parker J, Ham L, Lie JT, Groeneveld-van Beek EA, Melles GR. Bowman layer transplantation to reduce and stabilize progressive, advanced keratoconus. *Ophthalmology.* 2015;122:909-917.

Please see videos on the accompanying website at
www.healio.com/books/DALKvideos

8

Intraoperative Optical Coherence Tomography in DALK

Kristin E. Hirabayashi, MD and Charles C. Lin, MD

Deep anterior lamellar keratoplasty (DALK) is an excellent surgical option in patients with corneal pathology that have preserved endothelial function, such as keratoconus, stromal scarring due to infectious and noninfectious conditions, and corneal dystrophies. Compared to penetrating keratoplasty (PK), it offers a variety of immunological and mechanical advantages. Preservation of the host endothelium decreases the risk of allograft rejection and can also lessen the reliance on postoperative topical steroids.[1,2] This can be a critical advantage in patients who are phakic, steroid responders, or poorly compliant. DALK has also been shown to have less endothelial cell loss after surgery compared to PK.[1,3-6] There are obvious safety advantages to avoiding the open-sky component of PK, especially mitigating the risk of suprachoroidal hemorrhage. Furthermore, DALK offers the potential for faster visual rehabilitation as sutures can be removed earlier in the postoperative course compared to PK.[5] Finally, in terms of graft survival, DALK has been shown to have fewer rejection episodes compared to PK.[1,7]

Although DALK carries significant advantages over PK, the technical challenges of DALK have limited more widespread adoption. Prior studies have reported mixed conclusions regarding the visual outcomes of DALK compared to PK and surgeon experience plays a significant role.[1,2,4,7-9] The American Academy of Ophthalmology does recommend DALK as a preferred technique.[10] Baring Descemet's membrane (DM), or leaving minimal residual posterior stroma, underlies successful DALK surgery. In fact, leaving a residual stromal thickness of 20 μm or less correlates with superior visual outcomes.[11,12] Intraoperative optical coherence tomography (iOCT) can help achieve this goal by providing visualization of cross-sectional anatomy to guide cornea stromal dissection.

Jacob S, ed. *Mastering DALK: A Video Textbook on Deep Anterior Lamellar Keratoplasty* (pp 93-103).

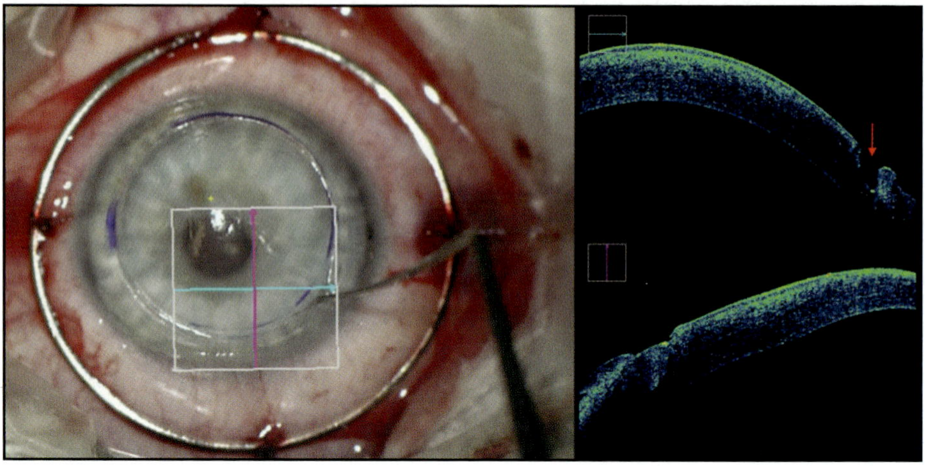

Figure 8-1. A microcyclodialysis spatula partially opens the trephination groove to reveal a penetration depth approximately two-thirds of the corneal stroma (red arrow), best appreciated on the horizontal section of the OCT cross-hair image.

Intraoperative Optical Coherence Tomography Applications for DALK

OCT is a non-contact imaging modality that uses light to discriminate fine details in anatomical structures on the order of microns. iOCT enables a real-time anatomical cross-sectional view of the cornea, which can provide invaluable information to a surgeon performing DALK. There are currently 2 iOCT models on the market. First, the Zeiss Rescan (Carl Zeiss Meditech) has an OCT built into the operating microscope, and the OCT images can be viewed on an attached screen or through a heads-up display in the oculars. It is a spectral domain OCT that uses light with a wavelength of 840 nanometers and has an axial resolution of 5.5 µm in tissue. It provides real-time high resolution 1-line, 5-lines, and cross-hair images and can capture 1-line, 5-lines, and cube scans. Second, the Leica EnFocus OCT (Leica Microsystems) comes in 2 forms: Ultra-HD OCT and Ultra-Deep OCT. The Ultra-HD OCT uses light with a wavelength of 860 nanometers and has an axial resolution of 4 micrometers, and the Ultra-Deep OCT uses light with a wavelength of 880 nanometers and has an axial resolution of 9 micrometers. It can perform line, rectangular, annular, and radial scans. Similar to the Rescan OCT, it is integrated into an operating microscope, and the OCT images can be viewed through the oculars.

iOCT may be helpful in several steps of DALK surgery (Video 8-1). First, OCT can image the depth of the initial trephination. Using preoperative pachymetry, the trephination depth can be targeted to the deep stroma with caution to avoid premature perforation. iOCT allows real-time visualization of the depth of penetration and can help the surgeon determine if deeper trephination is needed[13] (Figure 8-1).

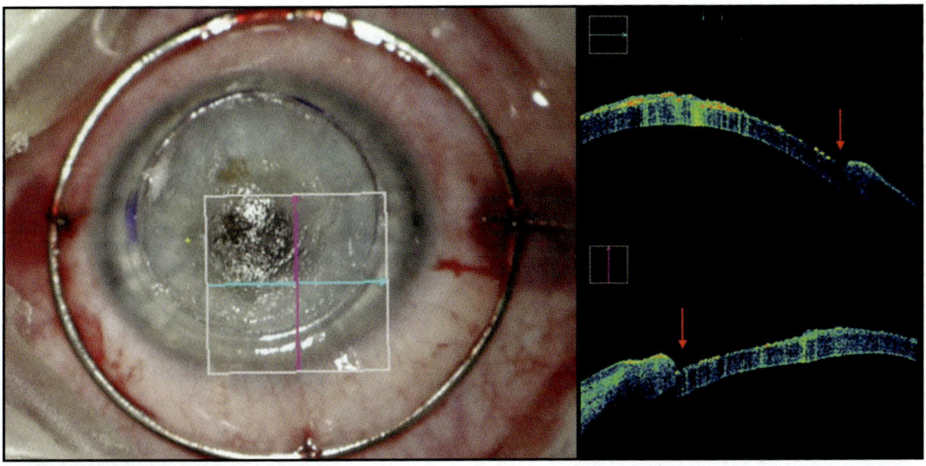

Figure 8-2. At the trephine edge (red arrow), the iOCT image shows that the anterior one-third of the stroma has been removed.

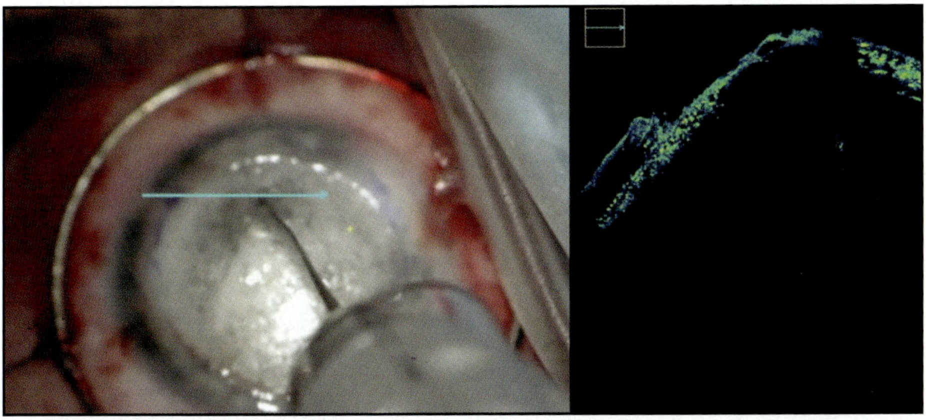

Figure 8-3. The view through the operating microscope on the left shows severe stromal emphysema that makes assessing the thickness of the residual stroma challenging. The OCT image shows residual posterior stroma of varying thickness with intrastromal bubbles.

Following removal of the anterior stroma, OCT images can be used to assess thickness of the residual stromal bed, a task that is more difficult to ascertain with the usual en face microscope perspective (Figure 8-2). This can be particularly useful in cases with decreased visualization (Video 8-2), such as a stromal scar or stromal emphysema (Figure 8-3), as well as in severely ectatic keratoconic eyes with significant apical thinning and a higher perforation risk. It may also be useful in the Jacob modified technique of primary management of acute hydrops with pre-Descemetic DALK (described in detail elsewhere in this book) to determine depth of dissection through the edematous hydrops tissue.[14,15]

A critical step in DALK surgery is attaining a deep stromal tunnel prior to attempting a big bubble air injection. Regardless of whether the big bubble is

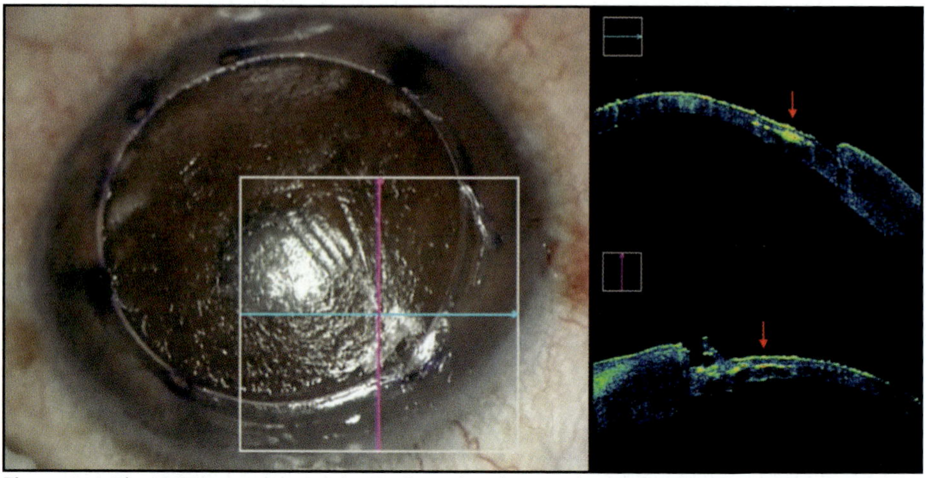

Figure 8-4. The iOCT image locates the Fogla probe–dissected tunnel within the anterior half of the residual stromal bed (red arrow).

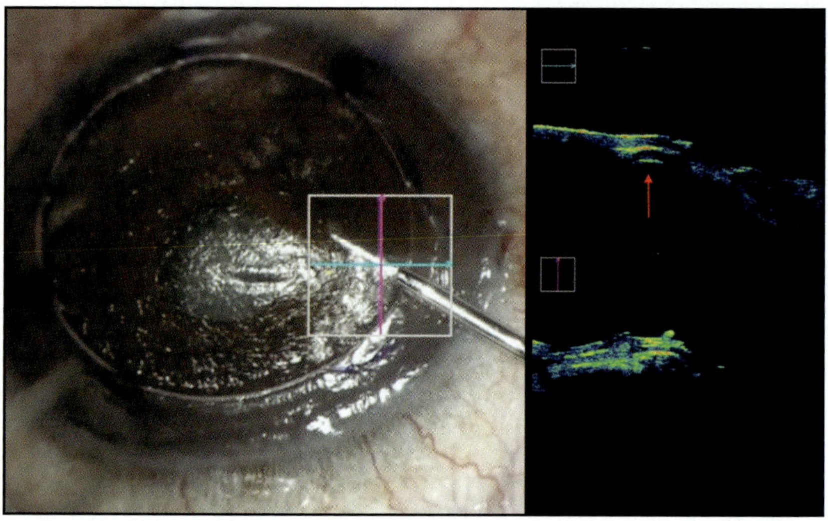

Figure 8-5. The Fogla probe is used to create a deeper stromal tunnel. While metallic artifact partially obscures the OCT image, the probe is located in the posterior half of the residual stromal bed (red arrow), which improves the probability of achieving a big bubble.

attempted with a needle or Fogla cannula, positioning the tunnel in the deep posterior stroma increases the chance of a successful big bubble. Prior reports indicate that placement of the cannula less than 100 μm from DM maximizes the chance of successful big bubble formation.[16,17] A superficial placement, as shown in Figure 8-4, often results in stromal emphysema, which may impair further visualization. Real-time OCT imaging during stromal tunnel creation can provide guidance for a more posterior position of the needle or cannula while preventing excessive tunneling and perforation (Figure 8-5 and Video 8-1).

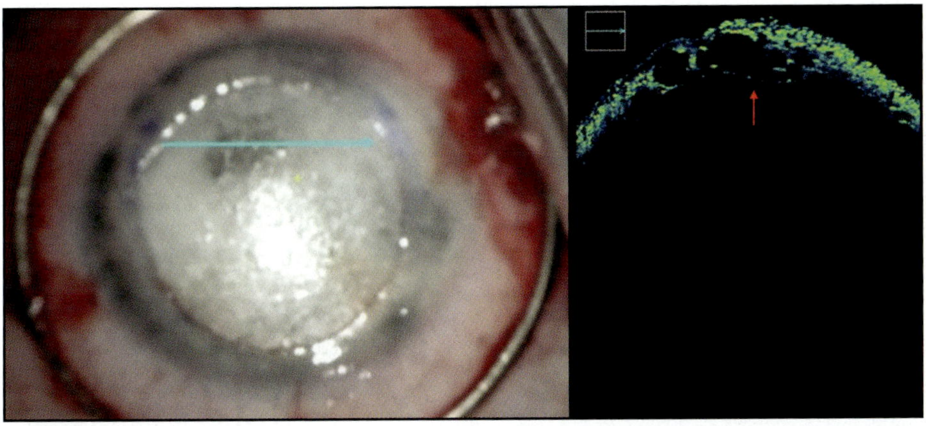

Figure 8-6. Significant intrastromal emphysema obscures the surgeon's view through the operating microscope, hindering evaluation of a successful big bubble. However, the high-resolution iOCT 1-line scan reveals a partial big bubble with an intact DM (red arrow).

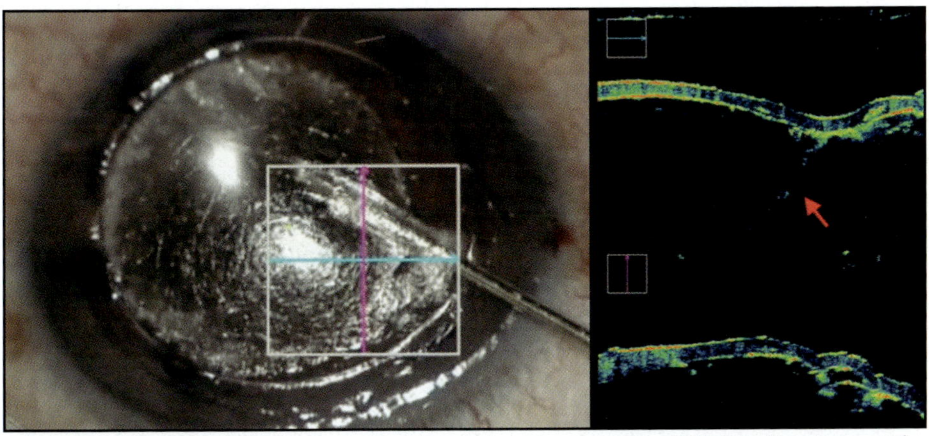

Figure 8-7. OCT confirms the presence of a big bubble with separation of DM from the stroma at the edge of the big bubble (red arrow).

In most cases, attainment of the big bubble is fairly obvious; however, uncertainty may arise when there is only a small big bubble, or when significant overlying stromal emphysema obscures visualization. In these cases, iOCT can help evaluate for the presence of a big bubble (Figure 8-6 and Video 8-2). Imaging the entire stroma–big bubble–Descemet membrane complex may require zooming out to increase the OCT field of view, especially in the case of a large big bubble with significant anterior-posterior height. Alternatively, focusing at the edge of the big bubble can identify separation of DM from stroma (Figure 8-7).

When a big bubble has not been achieved, iOCT can be used to guide manual dissection. In this case, the primary benefit of OCT is visualization of the extent of the remaining stromal tissue, a challenging task using the view from the operating microscope (Figure 8-8).[18] A cautious layer-by-layer approach to stromal removal can

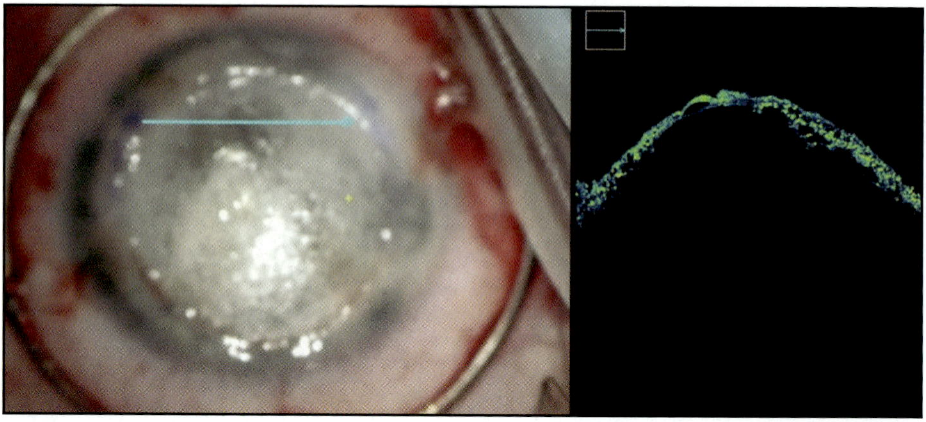

Figure 8-8. Layer-by-layer manual stromal dissection has been performed, but significant intrastromal emphysema limits an accurate assessment of residual stromal thickness with the operating microscope view on the left. In contrast, the iOCT image clearly shows a mild amount of residual stroma with what appears to be a small big bubble separation of DM.

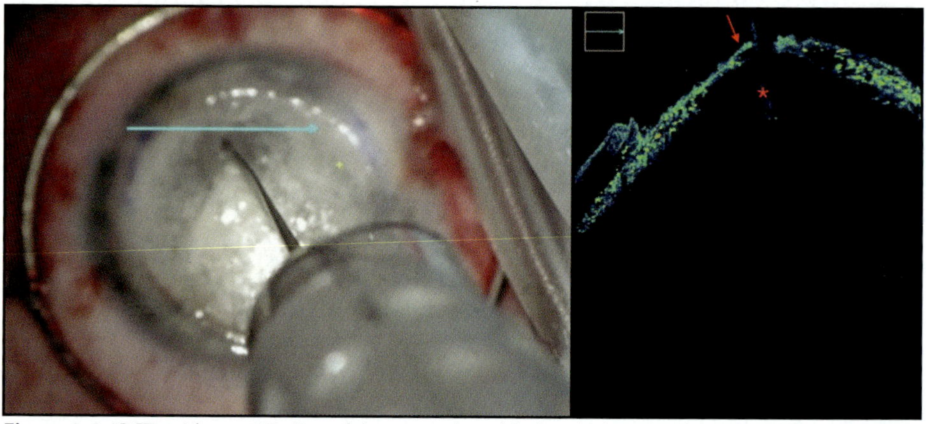

Figure 8-9. iOCT guides positioning of the super sharp blade, which casts a linear metallic artifact (red asterisk), over the small big bubble separating DM (red arrow).

be performed more safely under OCT guidance (Video 8-2). Additional attempts at the big bubble may be tried, but if none are successful the mini bubbles present in the stromal emphysema can be nicked open to facilitate deeper lamellar dissection with scissors (Figure 8-9).[19] This process can be repeated until DM is reached. The depth and proximity to DM of these mini bubbles can be visualized with iOCT, thus guiding additional dissection.

In the case of a perforation, iOCT can locate the perforation and the extent of the tear, critical information that guides further operative strategy (Video 8-3). Perforations are generally visible using a conventional microscope, but when residual overlying stroma is present, OCT can enhance visualization (Figure 8-10). The surgeon may choose to convert to a PK in the presence of a large central macroperforation

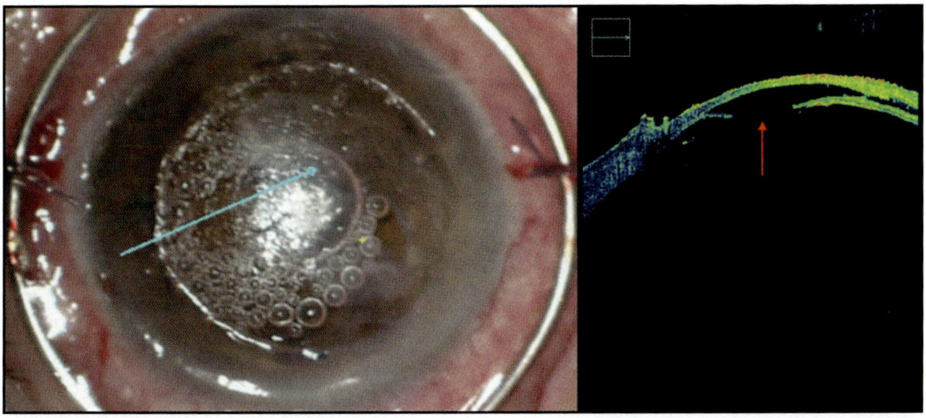

Figure 8-10. Numerous tiny air bubbles in the anterior chamber surround a larger air bubble, which appears to be a successful big bubble. However, iOCT shows that there is, in fact, a perforation as evidenced by the break in DM (red arrow).

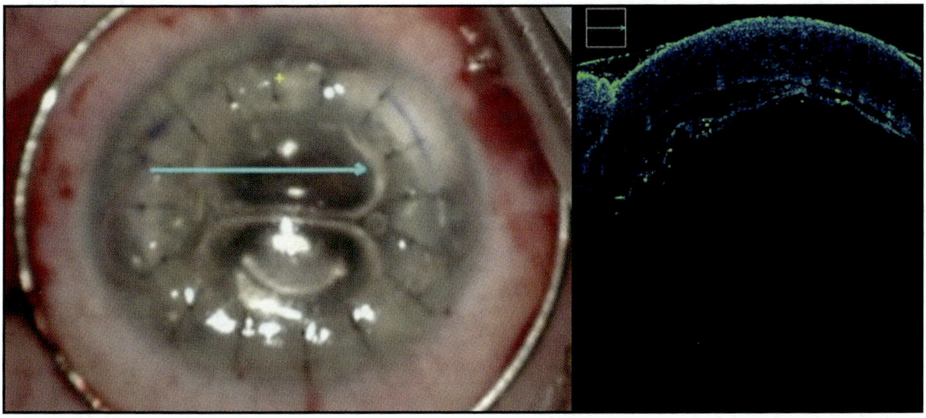

Figure 8-11. Following placement of the DALK donor graft, OCT shows moderate interface fluid with a partial intracameral air bubble.

but attempt to salvage the DALK for a peripheral macroperforation or small central microperforation. For the latter, a manual layer-by-layer stromal dissection approach can be employed, aided by iOCT guidance as previously described. Leaving more residual posterior stroma in the area of the perforation is advisable and OCT images can help the surgeon determine how aggressive to be with stromal dissection.

After the donor graft is sutured in place, iOCT imaging may confirm apposition of the graft and DM. There is often minimal interface fluid, which is inconsequential, as it rapidly self-resolves. If there is significant interface fluid as seen in Figure 8-11, then additional intracameral air can be injected to promote better apposition (Figure 8-12). However, if a perforation occurred, especially a macroperforation, iOCT images provide dynamic visualization of areas of Descemet's detachment. This can be managed with intracameral air injection to seal the perforation and tamponade

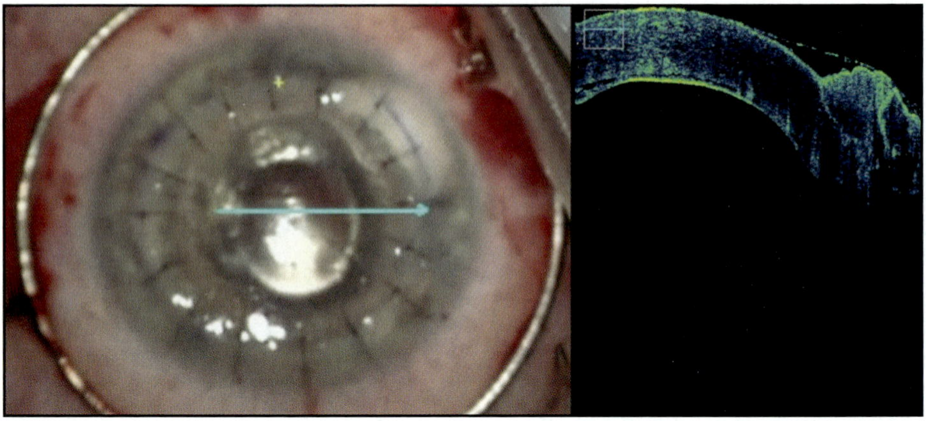

Figure 8-12. An injection of a larger intracameral air bubble mostly resolves the interface fluid, as evidenced by OCT.

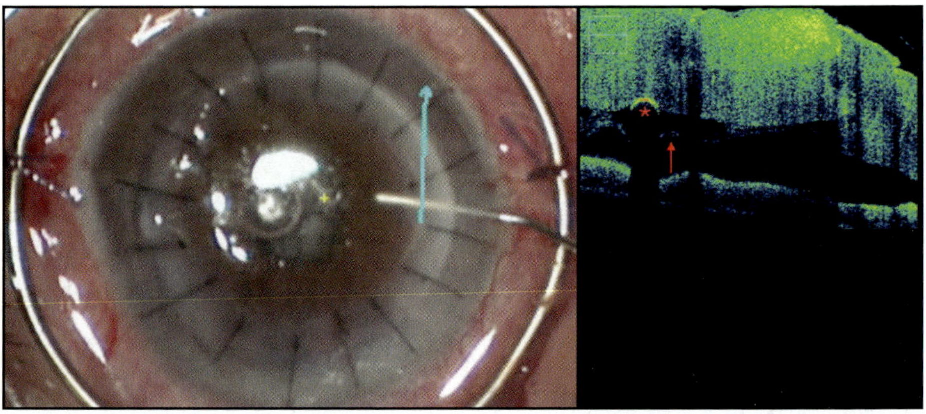

Figure 8-13. In this anatomically very narrow-angle, phakic eye, a cannula is placed to inject an intracameral air bubble to promote attachment of DM to the DALK graft. iOCT reveals that the cannula (red asterisk) is, in fact, in the interface between DM (red arrow) and the donor graft.

DM against the donor graft. iOCT can also help confirm that the cannula is properly positioned in the anterior chamber before injection to ensure that air is not injected into the interface between DM and the donor graft. This is less of a problem with peripheral and short paracenteses but can be more of a challenge with long paracenteses or in cases with significant stromal emphysema impeding the view. Figure 8-13 shows a phakic eye with an anatomically very narrow angle for which cannula placement presented a unique challenge. Initial placement of the cannula appeared to be in the correct location with direct microscopic visualization, but OCT revealed that the cannula was actually in the interface (Video 8-3). An adjacent, peripheral, more vertical paracentesis was created to allow for positioning the cannula in the correct location posterior to DM, permitting air injection into the anterior chamber

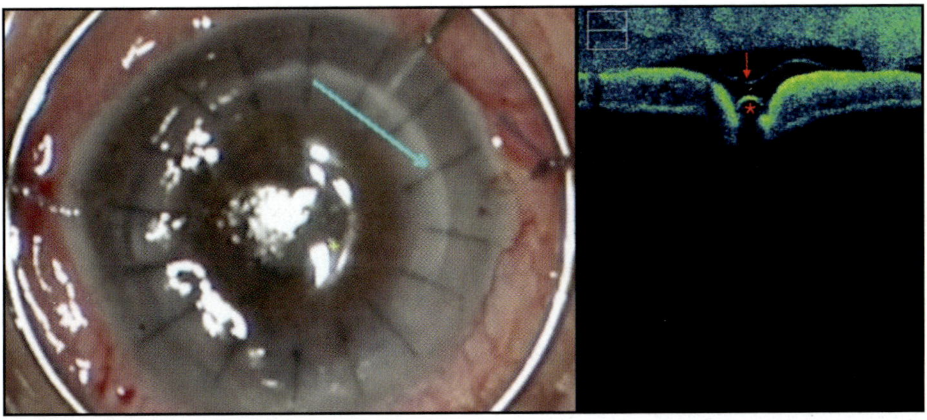

Figure 8-14. The cannula is placed through an adjacent paracentesis, and OCT shows that the cannula (asterisk) is in the correct location, posterior to Descemet's membrane (red arrow) and on top of the iris within a very shallow, nearly flat anterior chamber.

(Figure 8-14). If anatomic apposition is not apparent with iOCT, additional air injection may be necessary to pressurize the anterior chamber.

Conclusion

DALK is the preferred surgery for corneal stromal pathology yet it is a more technically challenging, time-consuming surgery with a steep learning curve compared to PK. Knowledge and recognition of corneal cross-sectional anatomy and depth is invaluable for lamellar keratoplasty, particularly DALK surgery, and underlies the power of iOCT. The high-resolution, real-time imaging provided by iOCT makes it an advantageous tool for surgeons performing DALK. iOCT provides real-time visualization of corneal depth and anatomy, which can assist the corneal surgeon in many steps of DALK surgery, including trephination, removal of the anterior stroma, stromal tunnel dissection, and big bubble attempts. One of the most critical and challenging steps of DALK is attaining a deep stromal dissection plane prior to attempting a big bubble. iOCT displays the stromal tunnel depth, guiding its placement and allowing for more consistent big bubble formation. The benefits of iOCT are particularly evident in challenging cases with impaired visualization, failed big bubble, and cornea perforation that may require manual stromal dissection.

REFERENCES

1. Liu H, Chen Y, Wang P, et al. Efficacy and safety of deep anterior lamellar keratoplasty vs. penetrating keratoplasty for keratoconus: a meta-analysis. *PLoS One*. 2015;10(1):e0113332.
2. Keane M, Coster D, Ziaei M, Williams K. Deep anterior lamellar keratoplasty versus penetrating keratoplasty for treating keratoconus. *Cochrane Database Syst Rev*. 2014;(7):CD009700.
3. Ku BI, Hsieh YT, Hu FR, Wan IJ, Chen WL, Hou YC. Endothelial cell loss in penetrating keratoplasty, endothelial keratoplasty, and deep anterior lamellar keratoplasty. *Taiwan J Ophthalmol*. 2017;7(4):199-204.
4. Reinhart WJ, Musch DC, Jacobs DS, Lee WB, Kaufman SC, Shtein RM. Deep anterior lamellar keratoplasty as an alternative to penetrating keratoplasty: a report by the American Academy of Ophthalmology. *Ophthalmology*. 2011;118(1):209-218.
5. Trimarchi F, Poppi E, Klersy C, Piacentini C. Deep lamellar keratoplasty. *Ophthalmologica*. 2001;215(6):389-393.
6. van Dooren BT, Mulder PG, Nieuwendaal CP, Beekhuis WH, Melles GR. Endothelial cell density after deep anterior lamellar keratoplasty (Melles technique). *Am J Ophthalmol*. 2004;137(3):397-400.
7. Kasbekar SA, Jones MN, Ahmad S, Larkin DF, Kaye SB; Ocular Tissue Advisory Group (audit study 15). Corneal transplant surgery for keratoconus and the effect of surgeon experience on deep anterior lamellar keratoplasty outcomes. *Am J Ophthalmol*. 2014;158(6):1239-1246.
8. Akdemir MO, Kandemir B, Sayman IB, Selvi C, Kamil Dogan O. Comparison of contrast sensitivity and visual acuity between deep anterior lamellar keratoplasty and penetrating keratoplasty in patients with keratoconus. *Int J Ophthalmol*. 2012;5(6):737-741.
9. Cohen AW, Goins KM, Sutphin JE, Wandling GR, Wagoner MD. Penetrating keratoplasty versus deep anterior lamellar keratoplasty for the treatment of keratoconus. *Int Ophthalmol*. 2010;30(6):675-681.
10. Reinhart WJ, Musch DC, Jacobs DS, Lee WB, Kaufman SC, Shtein RM. Deep anterior lamellar keratoplasty as an alternative to penetrating keratoplasty a report by the American Academy of Ophthalmology. *Ophthalmology*. 2011;118(1):209-218
11. Rama P, Knutsson KA, Razzoli G, Matuska S, Viganò M, Paganoni G. Deep anterior lamellar keratoplasty using an original manual technique. *Br J Ophthalmol*. 2013;97(1):23-27.
12. Ardjomand N, Hau S, McAlister JC, et al. Quality of vision and graft thickness in deep anterior lamellar and penetrating corneal allografts. *Am J Ophthalmol*. 2007;143(2):228-235.
13. Steven P, Le Blanc C, Lankenau E, et al. Optimising deep anterior lamellar keratoplasty (DALK) using intraoperative online optical coherence tomography (iOCT). *Br J Ophthalmol*. 2014;98(7):900-904.
14. Jacob S, Narasimhan S, Agarwal A, Sambath J, Umamaheshwari G, Saijimol AI. Primary modified predescemetic deep anterior lamellar keratoplasty in acute corneal hydrops. *Cornea*. 2018; 37(10):1328-1333.

15. Jacob S. Primary predescemetic DALK for acute hydrops Soosan Jacob with audio [video]. YouTube. https://www.youtube.com/watch?v=5ZeAXOmVDJw. Published June 14, 2018. Accessed September 27, 2018.
16. Pasricha ND, Shieh C, Carrasco-Zevallos OM, et al. Needle depth and big-bubble success in deep anterior lamellar keratoplasty: an ex vivo microscope-integrated OCT study. *Cornea.* 2016;35(11):1471-1477.
17. Scorcia V, Busin M, Lucisano A, Beltz J, Carta A, Scorcia G. Anterior segment optical coherence tomography-guided big-bubble technique. *Ophthalmology.* 2013;120(3):471-476.
18. De Benito-Llopis L, Mehta JS, Angunawela RI, Ang M, Tan DT. Intraoperative anterior segment optical coherence tomography: a novel assessment tool during deep anterior lamellar keratoplasty. *Am J Ophthalmol.* 2014;157(2):334-341.
19. Anwar DS, Kruger MM, Mootha VV. Blunt scissors stromal dissection technique for deep anterior lamellar keratoplasty. *Clin Ophthalmol.* 2014;8:1849-1854.

Please see videos on the accompanying website at
www.healio.com/books/DALKvideos

9

Primary Pre-Descemetic DALK in Acute Corneal Hydrops and Non–Big Bubble DALK in Older Patients

Soosan Jacob, MS, FRCS, DNB, MNAMS and Areeckal Incy Saijimol, BSc

Primary Pre-Descemetic DALK in Acute Corneal Hydrops

Acute corneal hydrops results from a spontaneous tear in the Descemet's membrane (DM) occurring in patients with advanced keratoconus. Aqueous seepage into the stroma through the tear results in a symptomatic patient with sudden decrease in vision. Conventional treatment for acute hydrops was medical management and, more recently, has consisted of intracameral gas (air, C_3F_8, SF_6, or C_2F_6). Though the acute hydrops generally resolves with these measures, it heals with the formation of a scar. The flattening caused by this scar formation can result in improvement in contact lens tolerance. Scarring may also result in improvement in visual acuity with peripherally located scars, albeit with disadvantages of the need for special and expensive contact lenses, limited hours of contact lens wear, poor vision in non-contact lens hours, poor contact lens fit and consequent complications, such as apical touch, apical scarring, and infectious keratitis. However, because it is often difficult to predict the location where scarring will develop or its extent, conventional treatment carries the risk of a scar developing in the visual axis that can impair vision. Many of these patients, therefore, ultimately require a secondary procedure either in the form of a pre-Descemetic deep anterior lamellar keratoplasty (PD-DALK) for

Jacob S, ed. *Mastering DALK: A Video Textbook on Deep Anterior Lamellar Keratoplasty* (pp 105-113).

peripheral scarring or a penetrating graft for centrally located scars.[1-14] The author (SJ) has described her technique of modified primary PD-DALK in acute corneal hydrops in a series of cases as immediate primary management modality at the time of presentation[15,16] to avoid post-hydrops scarring while providing visual, optical, topographic, structural, and biomechanical improvement while decreasing, and often avoiding, contact lens dependence as well as avoiding scar formation.

Clinical Examination and Investigations

Slit lamp examination of an eye with acute hydrops shows epithelial microcystic edema, stromal edema and swelling, intrastromal cyst/clefts, and conjunctival hyperemia. Careful examination may reveal the margins of the tear in some cases. Vision and intraocular pressure should be checked. Anterior segment optical coherence tomography (ASOCT) may be used to determine the corneal pachymetry, the extent of the tear along both the longest and shortest dimensions and location of the tear, as well as the amount of stroma over the tear. Topography of the involved eye may not be possible, but topography of the other eye may show evidence of keratoconus. In the absence of the ability to see the fundus clearly, an ultrasound evaluation of the posterior segment should be done.

Technique

The important surgical considerations to be understood for attaining a successful outcome are the following:

- The Descemet's tear is a weak point and should not be stressed mechanically.
- Thin layers of pre-Descemetic tissue should be retained over the tear in order to avoid opening the anterior chamber.
- In certain eyes with extensive thinning and hydrops, there may be very thin residual stroma over the break. In these cases, pressure from trephination of the cornea should be avoided.

Peribulbar block is used for cooperative patients. Intravenous sedation may be given. The desired diameter of the host bed is estimated by caliper. Depending on the structural integrity of the cornea, a decision is made as to whether a partial-thickness trephination of the cornea is possible. A partial-thickness trephination is performed in cases where the globe offers sufficient counter pressure. In cases with severe thinning and insufficient stroma over the tear, an inked trephine is instead used to mark the corneal surface. A sharp bevel up crescent dissector is then used to deepen this groove. A 26-gauge needle bent with its bevel up (instead of bevel down, as in big bubble DALK) is then mounted on a 1 mL syringe and used to inject air gently at multiple quadrants. The needle is inserted tangentially around the break at multiple spots and air is injected slowly in a graded manner in small aliquots around the tear, as well as other areas of the cornea, avoiding acute build-up of air pressure. The anterior stroma is then debulked with a blunt crescent blade using the emphysematous cornea as a guide to depth of dissection. An air bubble is then injected into the anterior chamber and deeper dissection is performed circumferentially from all

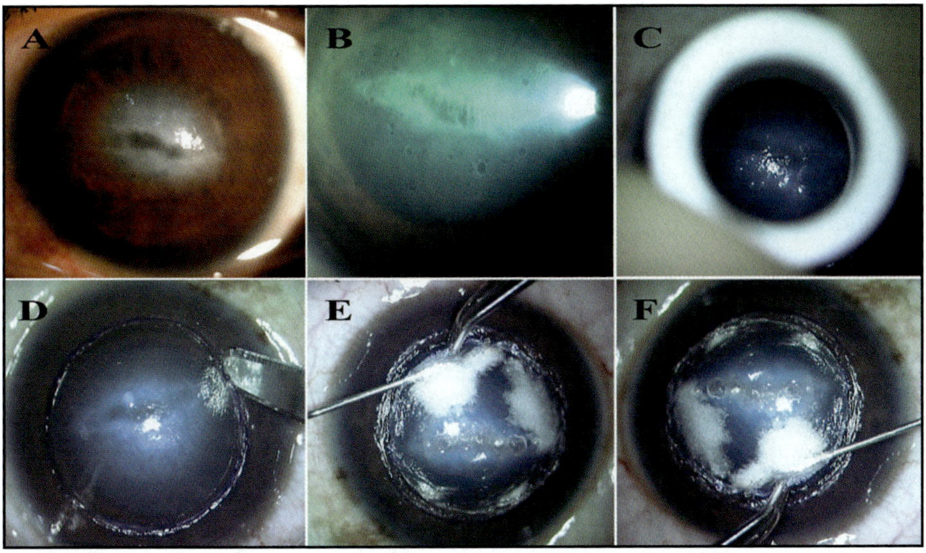

Figure 9-1. (A) Acute corneal hydrops. (B) Tear in DM seen better with endoilluminator. (C) Partial-thickness trephination done. (D) Groove is deepened with a crescent dissector. (E, F) A bevel up 26-gauge needle on a 1-mL syringe is inserted tangentially directed away from the ruptured DM. Surrounding cornea is made emphysematous using small aliquots of air directed away from the break.

sides starting from the periphery and working carefully towards the center using the Melles technique. The central undissected stroma is removed at the end dissecting carefully over the area of break. Minimal stroma is intentionally retained over the tear in order to retain a closed anterior chamber. If at any point the anterior chamber is soft or shallow, air is injected into the anterior chamber through the small paracentesis. Finally, a same-sized graft trephined from a donor corneoscleral rim from which DM has been removed, is sutured onto the host bed. Air is finally injected into the anterior chamber to tamponade the DM tear (Figures 9-1 and 9-2 and Video 9-1).

Discussion

In a case series of 11 patients presenting with acute hydrops, the author has successfully performed PD-DALK using the aforementioned modifications in all cases without any corneal perforations. Though air entered the anterior chamber through the DM tear in many cases, it did not enlarge the tear in any case in our series. All corneas healed without scarring over the area of the Descemetic tear, which is a major advantage (Figures 9-3 and 9-4). This is unlike the healing by scarring that is generally seen after conventional management techniques (Figure 9-5A). It can take up to 2 to 3 months for healing post-hydrops, and it is probable that this prolonged period of persistent edema provokes increased inflammation that results in healing by scarring. A secondary PD-DALK done for healed hydrops also often cannot attain complete scar removal and residual scar is common and can be a disadvantage when in the visual axis (Figure 9-5B). Intracameral gas keeps the torn Descemet's edges

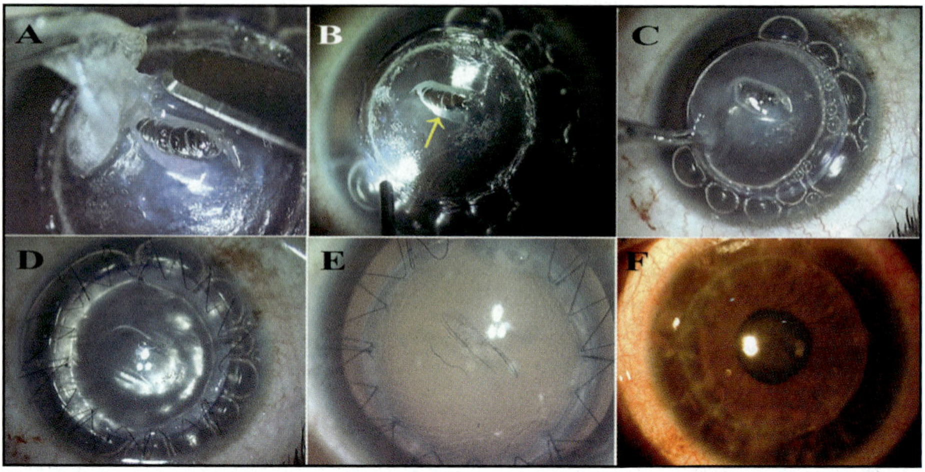

Figure 9-2. (A) The overlying stroma is dissected using the emphysematous stroma as a guide for the dissection plane. Deeper layer, if present, is removed by careful manual dissection of the deeper stromal layers using a blunt crescent dissector with the Melles technique. (B) Dissection completed. Host cornea seen after pre-Descemetic dissection. An elliptical Descemet's break is seen (arrow) with minimal retained overlying intact pre-Descemetic stroma. The anterior chamber is well-maintained with no escape of air. (C, D) Donor graft with DM stripped is sutured onto the host bed. (E, F) Clear graft and visual axis seen at 6 months postoperative. Torn, scrolled edges of the DM tear is seen with clear overlying stroma.

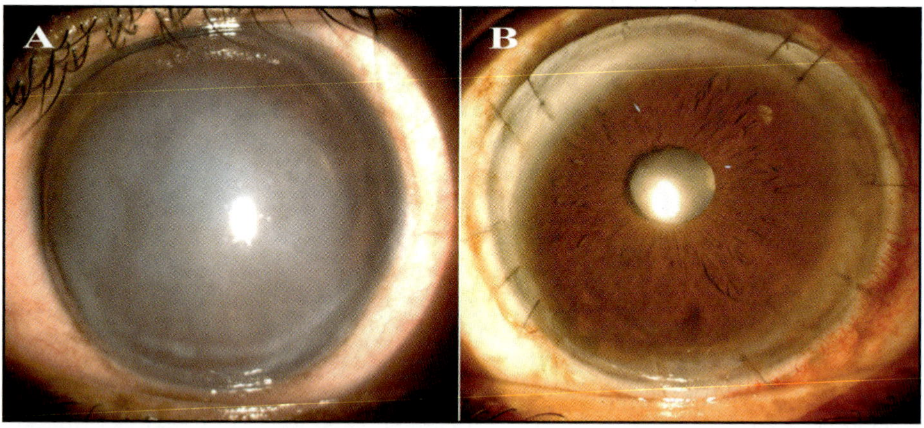

Figure 9-3. (A) Preoperative picture of patient 1 showing Grade 3 acute corneal hydrops. (B) Postoperative picture showing clear graft.

widely separated under an ectatic cornea, whereas a primary DALK brings the torn edges closer with decreased separation. As the edema has a fast resolution following primary PD-DALK, none of the cases in our series showed scarring in the area of Descemet's tear and the overlying stroma remained clear in all patients. Maintenance of clarity in the absence of endothelial cells in the area of tear is because of the ability of the adjacent endothelial cells to maintain corneal deturgescence. Endothelial cells may also enlarge and slide over to cover the defect, though confocal microscopy

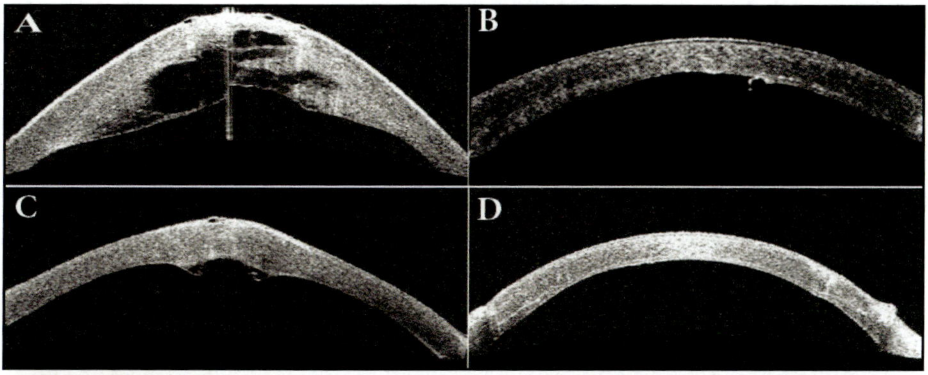

Figure 9-4. (A) Preoperative ASOCT showing DM tear, large clefts, and stromal thinning. (B) Postoperative ASOCT showing area with defect in DM with overlying non-edematous cornea. A pre-Descemetic plane of dissection is seen. (C, D) Another case showing pre- and postoperative ASOCT.

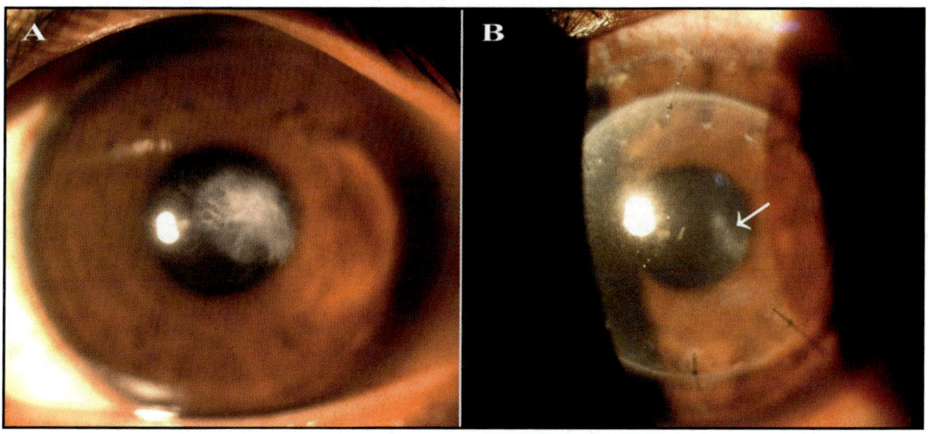

Figure 9-5. (A) Post-hydrops scarring when left to heal on its own or with other surgical interventions, such as air injection. (B) Residual scar remains even after secondary PD-DALK.

would be needed to prove this. This is similar to the stromal clarity that is maintained in the gap between the graft and the area of host Descemetic stripping following a DM-endothelial keratoplasty.

Conventional management that includes conservative management, intracameral isoexpansile gas injection,[1,2] compressive sutures along with gas injection,[6] penetrating keratoplasty (PK),[1,2] cyanoacrylate tissue adhesive with bandage contact lens,[7] and amniotic membrane transplantation with cauterization[8] all result in corneal scarring that is followed by a flattening with or without improvement in contact lens tolerance and sometimes decreased visual acuity in case of visual axis scars. Collagen cross-linking to stabilize the cornea is often not possible in these cases of advanced keratoconus because of pachymetry below the limits for safe cross-linking that precludes this procedure. A second stage DALK is therefore often required in many cases to improve vision, especially in contact lens intolerant patients.[9]

Leaving the acute hydrops patient to heal by scarring has several disadvantages. The patient has low visual acuity for a prolonged period together with risk of perforation in patients with extreme thinning.[9,10] Other techniques, such as pneumodescemetopexy, compression sutures, cyanoacrylate glue, thermokeratoplasty, and amniotic membrane grafting, also result in scarring requiring a secondary surgical intervention in the form of a PD-DALK or optical PK for visual axis scarring, visual rehabilitation, thinning, or ectasia. This requirement for 2 surgeries increases comorbidity, cost of treatment, and time required for treatment. The modifications described by the author for primary PD-DALK for acute corneal hydrops allows a single-staged treatment thereby having advantages of early visual and anatomic rehabilitation, while retaining the host endothelium.

Enlargement of the Descemetic tear is avoided in this technique by using a needle with bevel bent upward, by directing the needle tangentially away from the hydrops while injecting air and by injecting small aliquots of air at a time, monitoring the direction of creation of emphysema. Retaining minimum stroma above the DM tear prevents direct perforation into the anterior chamber. Tamponading the DM against the sutured graft with an air bubble in the anterior chamber allows closure of the DM tear by pneumodescemetopexy.[14]

Conclusion

Primary PD-DALK in acute hydrops helps close the DM break while avoiding the need for a second surgical procedure. The grafted cornea corrects the severe ectasia and thinning that may be seen in patients with severe keratoconus and hydrops while regularizing topography and improving vision. It retains the host DM and endothelium, avoids scarring secondary to hydrops, and provides early and rapid visual and anatomical rehabilitation. Surgery should be performed with care by an experienced surgeon, using the described technique.

Non–Big Bubble Pre-Descemetic DALK in Older Patients

While creating grafts for pre-Descemet's endothelial keratoplasty, it is known that a Type 2 big bubble forms more easily than a Type 1 big bubble in older donor corneas. This is because the attachment of the DM to the pre-Descemet's layer is stronger in younger corneas. The author (SJ) has noted in her personal experience that the incidence of obtaining a Type 2 big bubble is similarly higher when performing DALK in older patients. This is the reverse of what is seen in younger patients who have a greater incidence of a Type 1 big bubble forming on forceful injection of air.

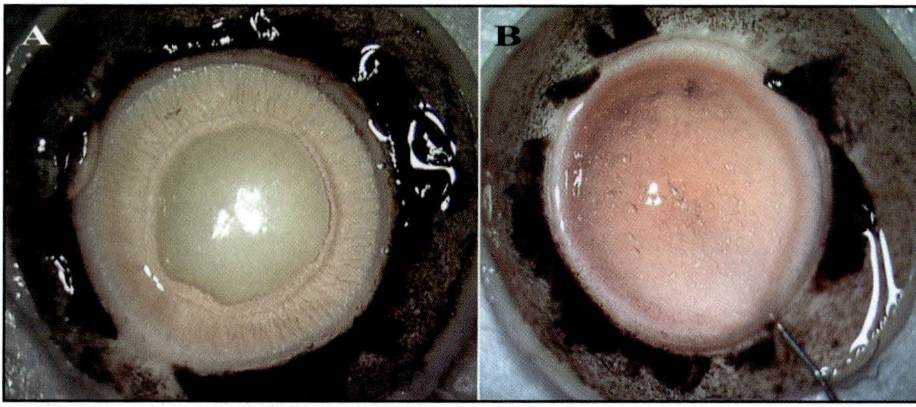

Figure 9-6. (A) Type 1 big bubble. (B) Type 2 big bubble.

Type 1 Versus Type 2 Big Bubble

Creation of a Type 2 big bubble while performing DALK is seen as a small area of Descemetic separation that starts from the periphery and enlarges, unlike a Type 1 big bubble that classically starts from the center and enlarges circumferentially. Well-defined borders with a circumferential emphysematous expanding ring and tough, elevated dome-shaped appearance of the Type 1 big bubble are not seen. The Type 2 big bubble, instead, is a more delicate looking bubble with sloping edges and a mildly elevated contour. The typical circumferential emphysematous expanding ring is not seen around the bubble and continued injection of air can cause the Type 2 big bubble to rupture with a resultant Descemetic tear. It is therefore important to identify this type of bubble as soon as it forms to avoid injecting further air that could expand it with resultant risk of rupture (Figure 9-6 and Video 9-2).

Surgical Technique

It is important to try to avoid this bubble from forming. With advancing age of the patient, it is impossible to predict which type of big bubble will be formed with the standard technique and the chances of a Type 2 big bubble are higher, so the author (SJ) prefers to use her modified non–big bubble technique of DALK in patients above the age of 40. This is done using some of the principles mentioned previously in primary PD-DALK for acute hydrops. Trephination is confined to 60% depth and air is then injected in a slow, controlled, graded manner with a 26-gauge needle bent with bevel facing up to induce tissue emphysema. Multiple puncture points are used, and small aliquots of air are injected at multiple spots to avoid creating a big bubble. Superficial stroma is then dissected using the emphysematous stroma as a guide to depth. A small paracentesis is created, and air is injected into the anterior chamber. Deeper layers of stroma are then dissected using the Melles technique using the reflex at the air-Descemetic interface as a guide. Once adequately deep dissection is performed, a donor graft stripped of its DM is sutured on to the host cornea (Video 9-3).

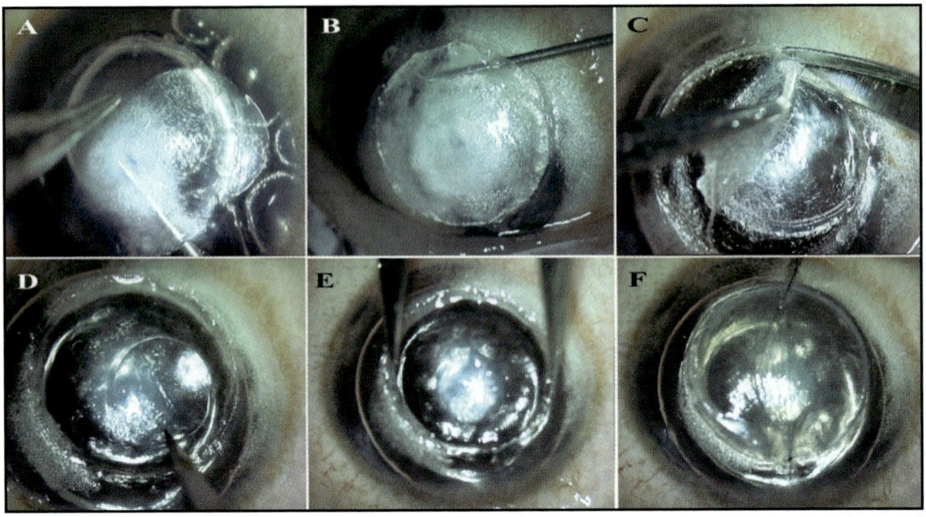

Figure 9-7. (A) Type 2 big bubble obtained during DALK in a 45-year-old patient. (B) Superficial stromal emphysema induced by injecting air. (C) Manual superficial stromal dissection done. (D, E) Type 2 big bubble punctured from stromal side to let out air. (F) Donor graft sutured into place.

Management of Type 2 Big Bubble

If a Type 2 big bubble does form, it is imperative to stop injecting further air and continue with a non–big bubble type of dissection as just described. Deroofing or applying a nick on the Type 2 big bubble from the stromal aspect decompresses it and PD-DALK can be continued with (Figure 9-7 and Video 9-2). In case there is a rupture of the Type 2 big bubble, further dissection should again be carried out using the non–big bubble dissection technique described by the author. Care should be taken to leave a few pre-Descemetic and stromal layers intact above the area of DM tear to avoid opening and collapse of the anterior chamber. The donor cornea is then sutured in place and air is injected into the anterior chamber to tamponade the DM tear against the overlying stroma. In case of a flapped tear of the DM, an anterior chamber connected to an air pump is inserted into the anterior chamber and a reverse Sinskey hook is used to gently reposition the torn DM in place against the overlying stroma.

References

1. Tuft SJ, Gregory WM, Buckley RJ. Acute corneal hydrops in keratoconus. *Ophthalmology.* 1994;101(10):1738-1744.
2. Sharma N, Maharana PK, Jhanji V, Vajpayee RB. Management of acute corneal hydrops in ectatic corneal disorders. *Curr Opin Ophthalmol.* 2012;23(4):317-323
3. Archila EA. Deep lamellar keratoplasty dissection of host tissue with intrastromal air injection. *Cornea.* 1984-1985;3:217-218.
4. Melles GR, Lander F, Rietveld FJ, Remeijer L, Beekhuis WH, Binder PS. A new surgical technique for deep stromal, anterior lamellar keratoplasty. *Br J Ophthalmol.* 1999;83:327-333.

5. Maharana PK, Sharma N, Vajpayee RB. Acute corneal hydrops in keratoconus *Indian J Ophthalmol.* 2013;61(8):461–464.
6. Rajaraman R, Singh S, Raghavan A, Karkhanis A. Efficacy and safety of intracameralperfluoropropane (C3F8) tamponade and compression sutures for the management of acute corneal hydrops. *Cornea.* 2009;28(3):317-320.
7. Aldave AJ, Mabon M, Hollander DA, McLeod SD, Spencer WH, Abbott RL. Spontaneous corneal hydrops and perforation in keratoconus and pellucid marginal degeneration. *Cornea.* 2003;22(2):169-174.
8. Wylegala E, Tarnawska D. Amniotic membrane transplantation with cauterization for keratoconus complicated by persistent hydrops in mentally retarded patients. *Ophthalmology.* 2006;113(4):561-564
9. Li S, Liu M, Wang Q, Wang T, Shi W. Lamellar keratoplasty following thermokeratoplasty in the treatment of acute corneal hydrops. *Am J Ophthalmol.* 2014;158(1):26-31.
10. Ch'ng SW, Pillai MB, Aazeem S, Tu KL. Acute corneal hydrops mimicking full thickness perforation. *BMJ Case Rep.* 2012;2012:bcr0120125496. doi: 10.1136/bcr.01.2012.5496
11. Sarnicola V, Toro P, Gentile D, Hannush SB. Descemetic DALK and predescemetic DALK: outcomes in 236 cases of keratoconus. *Cornea.* 2010;29(1):53-59.
12. Abdelkader A, Kaufman HE. Descemetic versus pre-Descemetic lamellar keratoplasty: clinical and confocal study. *Cornea.* 2011;30(11):1244-1252.
13. Nanavaty MA, Daya SM. Outcomes of deep anterior lamellar keratoplasty in keratoconic eyes with previous hydrops. *Br J Ophthalmol.* 2012;96(10):1304-1309.
14. Jacob S, Agarwal A, Chaudhry P, Narasimhan S, Chaudhry VN. A new clinico-tomographic classification and management algorithm for Descemet's membrane detachment. *Cont Lens Anterior Eye.* 2015;38(5):327-333.
15. Jacob S, Narasimhan S, Agarwal A, Sambath J, Umamaheshwari G, Saijimol AI. Primary modified predescemetic deep anterior lamellar keratoplasty in acute corneal hydrops. *Cornea.* 2018; 37(10):1328-1333.
16. Jacob S. Primary predescemetic DALK for acute hydrops Soosan Jacob with audio [video]. YouTube. https://www.youtube.com/watch?v=5ZeAXOmVDJw. Published June 14, 2018. Accessed September 27, 2018.

Please see videos on the accompanying website at
www.healio.com/books/DALKvideos

10

DALK in Complex Situations
Corneal Infections, Chemical Burns, and Others

Namrata Sharma, MD; Deepali Singhal, MD, DNB, FICO, FICO Cornea; Pranita Sahay, MD; and Prafulla Maharana, MD

Deep anterior lamellar keratoplasty (DALK) is a well-known surgical technique that involves excision of the pathological stroma until the Descemet's membrane (DM), leaving the original corneal endothelium intact.[1] This has been described as the *Descemetic DALK* (D-DALK). If, however, around 90% of the stroma is removed leaving behind a layer of posterior stroma, it is termed as *pre-Descemetic DALK* (PD-DALK).[1]

The major advantages as compared to penetrating keratoplasty (PK) include avoiding the complications associated with an open-sky surgery, a low-risk of graft rejection, less postoperative management, and optimal utilization of donor corneas in developing countries. All these advantages, especially the advantages of being a predominantly extraocular procedure, together with lack of endothelial rejection makes DALK a suitable procedure in difficult situations, like ocular surface diseases, infectious keratitis, and descmetocele.[1-3]

DALK in Corneal Infections

The mainstay of therapy of infective keratitis is medical management initially. Surgical management is required in instances of refractory cases, descemetocele, scleral extension, and corneal perforation.[4,5] To date, therapeutic PK has been the standard procedure for infective keratitis. However, it is associated with certain limitations, including high risk of graft failure because of recurrence (50% to 82%), endophthalmitis (ie, intraocular spread of infection during surgery), and a subsequent

Jacob S, ed. *Mastering DALK: A Video Textbook on Deep Anterior Lamellar Keratoplasty* (pp 115-126).

higher risk of graft rejection in subsequent optical grafts in these inflamed, often vascularized, high-risk eyes.[6] DALK has been tried as a surgical option in infective keratitis (termed as *therapeutic DALK* [T-DALK]) for cases of bacterial, fungal, viral, *Acanthamoeba* as well as *Microsporidia* keratitis.[4,6-10]

Indications

Infective keratitis involving the corneal stroma with sparing of the DM-endothelium complex and refractory to medical therapy is the main indication of T-DALK.

Contraindications

In the scenario of infective keratitis, DALK is contraindicated when there is full-thickness corneal involvement requiring PK, or in the presence of corneal perforation.

Advantages

The advantages of DALK over PK in case of infective keratitis include reduced risk of complications, such as endophthalmitis, endothelial graft rejection and subsequent failure, cataract, or glaucoma; reduced risk of complications associated with open-sky procedures; decreased requirement for prolonged use of steroids; and optimal utilization of donor corneas in developing countries. It helps healing by removing the infective focus, limiting the intraocular spread, and minimizing the risk of graft failure.

Preoperative Evaluation

A detailed ocular history is important, along with a meticulous slit lamp examination. Anterior and posterior segment examination should be completed along with measurement of intraocular pressure. Extent of stromal infiltration and the depth of involvement should be carefully noted. An anterior segment optical coherence tomography can also help in assessing the depth of stromal involvement. A detailed microbiological examination of corneal scraping is required to know the infective agent.

Surgical Technique

Various techniques have been described for DALK, such as the air- or viscoelastic-assisted techniques, Melles technique, hydrodelamination, big bubble and double bubble techniques, diamond knife–assisted manual dissection, and femtosecond-assisted DALK.[1] However, in cases of infective keratitis, the preferred techniques include big bubble DALK and manual layer-by-layer dissection.[4,6-10]

The big bubble technique leads to complete baring of DM (D-DALK), whereas manual dissection retains some of the posterior stroma (PD-DALK). The big bubble technique is preferred in cases with normal peripheral cornea as well as relatively uninvolved posterior stromal layer. This is also preferred in cases of fungal and *Acanthamoeba* keratitis due to higher chances of retention of the infective organism in posterior stromal layers.[4] Air injection should be avoided in cases with necrotic stroma, such as *Pseudomonas* keratitis.

Anesthesia

Informed consent for the surgery should be obtained. The surgery can be performed under local anesthesia, though general anesthesia may be preferred in children and uncooperative patients, as well as to avoid the risk of perforation of bare DM intraoperatively.

Host Bed Preparation

A modified form of the standard Anwar big bubble technique has been described in most clinical studies.[4,6-10] An 8.00- to 9.00-mm partial-thickness (60%) trephination with the Hanna corneal trephine (Moria) is performed. Manual anterior lamellar dissection of the anterior stroma is then done with a crescent blade (1.25 mm; Sharpoint) to a depth of approximately 50% of the corneal stroma. A 30-gauge needle attached to a 2-mL syringe and bent at 15° to 30° is advanced with bevel down into the paracentral corneal stroma. About 1 to 1.5 mL of sterilized air is injected into the posterior stroma until a big bubble is formed extending to the border of trephination. Residual stroma is then removed in quadrants, revealing bare DM. In cases with lack of big bubble formation, manual dissection is continued.

Donor Preparation

Full-thickness donor corneal tissues are used for transplantation. The donor cornea is punched from the endothelial side and is oversized by 0.25 mm. The donor DM and endothelium are stained with 0.06% trypan blue dye and then gently stripped using 0.12 mm non-toothed forceps or Merocel sponge (Beaver-Visitec International). This donor cornea is then sutured to the recipient with 16 interrupted 10-0 monofilament nylon sutures.

Viscoelastic-assisted DALK in descemetocele has been described by Sharma et al[11] in 12 cases of resolved microbial keratitis (Figure 10-1). All cases but 1 had significant improvement in visual acuity with clear grafts in 10 cases at last follow-up.

Postoperative Treatment

The postoperative medication consists of a topical antimicrobial agent tailored according to the causative organism.[3,4] In cases of bacterial infections, intensive, broad-spectrum antibiotic combinations are continued in the immediate postoperative period, together with systemic antibiotic cover, and gradually tapered if infection does not recur. Topical steroids for confirmed bacterial infections are usually initiated on postoperative day 3 or 4. For fungal infections, aggressive topical antifungal treatment in combination with oral fluconazole or voriconazole is given.

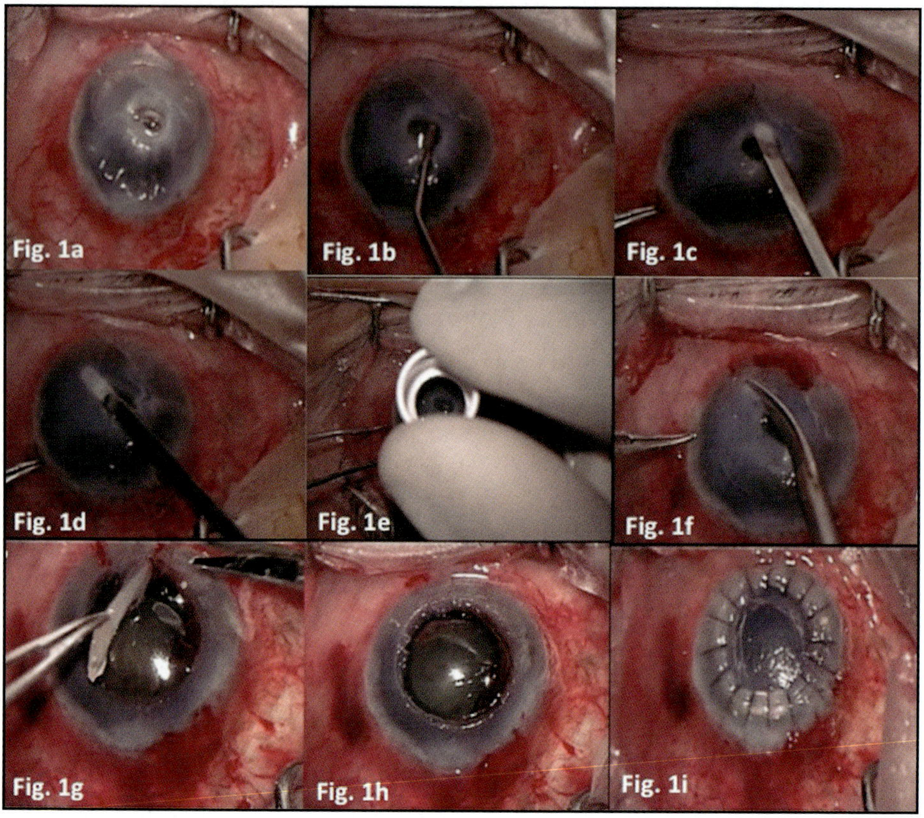

Figure 10-1. (A) A case of infective keratitis with central descemetocele. (B) 26-gauge cannula used to separate the plane between the clear DM, at the stromal edge in the area of the herniated DM. (C, D) The posterior stroma of the cornea above the membrane separated using a blunt spatula. (E) Partial-thickness trephination mark made with a disposable trephine. (F, G) The posterior stroma of the cornea above the membrane was excised using a blunt-tipped curved Vannas scissors by dividing into 4 quadrants, thus, baring the DM completely. (H) Exposure of bare DM. (I) Suturing of the donor corneal button to the host bed.

Antifungal treatment is maintained over a prolonged period of up to several months after surgery. Topical steroids are usually withheld for at least 1 to 2 weeks after surgery. Topical cyclosporine (0.5%) can be used in the early postoperative period as a steroid-sparing agent and for its potential antifungal effect. For *Acanthamoeba* keratitis, patients are maintained on multiple medications, including combination of polyhexamethylbiguanide, chlorhexidine, propamidine isethionate, and hexamidine, with or without topical steroids, for several weeks to months after surgery, with gradual tapering.[3,4]

Complications

The specific complications of DALK in infectious keratitis are included in the following sections.

Descemet's Membrane Perforation

The most important intraoperative complication of DALK is DM perforation.[3] Its incidence ranges between 4% and 20%, and this can occur at any step of surgery. A small perforation can be managed by intracameral injection of air and careful stromal dissection, while a large perforation requires conversion to PK. Anshu et al[4] reported intraoperative microperforation in 15.3% of cases but none required conversion to PK. Gao et al[12] noted perforation in 8.7% of cases of deep fungal keratitis. No intraoperative complication was seen in T-DALK done in a case of post-LASIK mycobacterial keratitis.[12] Sarnicola et al[8] reported 1 case (out of 11) with intraoperative microperforation during PD-DALK.

Pseudo Anterior Chamber

Anshu et al[4] reported postoperative DM detachment in 15.3% of cases that spontaneously resolved in most of the cases, and 1 was managed with intracameral air injection. Gao et al[12] noted perforation and double anterior chamber in 13% of cases of deep fungal keratitis.

Endophthalmitis

There was no case of T-DALK with postoperative endophthalmitis noted by Anshu et al[4] as compared to PK, which had an incidence of 5% to 10%.

Graft Rejection

Anshu et al[4] reported 10% to 15% incidence of graft rejection in PK group as compared to none in T-DALK group. Gao et al[12] noted stromal graft rejection in only 1 case (4.3%) of deep fungal keratitis during the first 3 months after surgery. No postoperative complication was seen in T-DALK done in a case of post-LASIK mycobacterial keratitis as well as in *Acanthamoeba* keratitis.[6,8,13]

Graft Failure

Late graft failure is reported to be in 1/26 cases in T-DALK as compared to 8/100 cases in PK group.[4]

Outcomes

Therapeutic Outcome

Anshu et al[4] reported recurrence in 4 patients (15.3%) in the T-DALK group compared with 12 (12%) in the PK group. The primary cause for eyes that developed a recurrence in the T-DALK group was bacterial (n = 2), fungal (n = 1), and *Acanthamoeba* (n = 1); all underwent surgery using the manual dissection technique. No recurrence of infection occurred in the T-DALK cases with total stromal removal. The T-DALK group also showed a trend toward better graft survival as compared to PK group (90% vs 78.4%).[4] Gao et al[12] reported a successful outcome of T-DALK in cases of deep fungal keratitis (4/5 of stromal involvement) with a recurrence in only 8.7% cases. No evidence of recurrence was seen in T-DALK done in a case of post-LASIK mycobacterial keratitis.[13]

Early T-DALK (within 30 to 60 days) has been considered a new approach to manage refractory/nonresponsive cases of *Acanthamoeba* keratitis. No episode of recurrence or failure was noted in these cases.[6,8] T-DALK has also been used successfully with no signs of recurrence or rejection for the treatment of microsporidial stromal keratitis.[10]

Visual Outcome

Anshu et al[4] reported a similar visual outcome in T-DALK and PK groups with a trend toward a better outcome in the DALK group. Gao et al[12] noted a significant improvement in visual acuity after T-DALK in deep fungal keratitis. A good visual outcome with an improvement from counting fingers to 20/50 was seen in a case of post-LASIK mycobacterial keratitis following T-DALK.[13] Significant improvement in best-corrected visual acuity (BCVA) was noted in cases of non-responsive *Acanthamoeba* keratitis post–T-DALK.[6,8]

DALK in Herpetic Stromal Keratitis

DALK has been evaluated in cases of active herpetic stromal keratitis (HSK), as well as quiescent and refractory cases.[9,14] It is a well-known fact that HSK can remain latent in the cornea leading to reactivation and increased risk of recurrence. PK is often required to eliminate most of the latent virus and thereby reduce the chances of recurrence. A recurrence rate of 25% in the first year and 44% in the second year has been reported with PK in HSK. The primary allograft rejection rate was 29% in the first year and 46% in the second.[15] In addition, the risk of graft failure in patients who underwent PK for HSK was higher than average, possibly due to the associated endothelial dysfunction.[16,17] Considering the various advantages of DALK over PK, it seems to be a safe and promising procedure for HSK, with a favorable visual outcome, graft survival rate, and lower endothelial cell loss.

Oral acyclovir prophylaxis started at least 1 month before surgery until at least 1 year after surgery plays an important role in reducing the rate of recurrence and rejection.[18] Various studies have shown encouraging outcomes with DALK as compared to PK in herpes simplex virus–related corneal scarring.[18-20] Awan et al[19] reported a 3-year graft survival rate of 83%, with a recurrence rate of 5%, and rejection rate of 33%, showing a better outcome as compared to PK. DALK using glycerin-preserved cornea has also shown to be an effective and safe therapy in refractory HSK (ie, HSK that recurred perennially for at least 3 years, with a shorter and shorter onset interval, exacerbated yearly with a poorly therapeutic effect).[14] However, a single study has evaluated the role of DALK in active HSK after amniotic membrane transplant and intravenous acyclovir.[9] They showed a graft survival rate of 86% with a significant improvement in vision and a recurrence of 18% of cases with active disease. Stromal rejection was seen in 2.3% cases only.[9]

Conclusion

With the advent of D-DALK procedures, such as the big bubble procedure, a higher chance of eradicating infection can be expected, with a lower recurrence rate of infections. It helps to avoid the complications of an open-sky procedure, reduces the risk of endophthalmitis, and preserves host endothelium thereby also reducing the chances of graft rejection and failure.

DALK IN CHEMICAL BURNS

The ocular surface, including both the corneal and conjunctival epithelium, is severely compromised following chemical injury. Limbal stem cells, which are the source for corneal epithelial cell regeneration, are also damaged. As a consequence, there is conjunctivalization, chronic inflammation, vascularization, persistent epithelial defects, and scarring of the cornea.[21] This results in symptoms of ocular discomfort and diminution of vision. Dense vascularization of the cornea predisposes to a high risk of graft rejection when conventional full-thickness keratoplasty is performed for these cases. Allogenic graft rejection rate as high as 57.7% has been reported in literature post-PK for chemical burn.[22] Thus, lamellar keratoplasty can improve long-term visual outcome in these cases by retaining the host endothelium and reducing the risk of immunologic endothelial graft rejection.

Surgical Technique

The major surgical challenge when performing DALK in these cases is the presence of corneal thinning, superficial vascularization of cornea leading to intra- and postoperative bleeding, and poor visibility due to the presence of corneal haze. Taking into consideration these factors, we recommend PD-DALK with a layer-by-layer manual dissection technique. An initial partial-thickness corneal trephination is done with a 7.7- or 8-mm corneal trephine to 75% corneal depth (Figure 10-2A). Lamellar dissection is then performed with the aid of a crescent blade while lifting the stromal tissue with the help of forceps (Figures 10-2B and 10-2C). At this step, it is important to maintain the plane of dissection. After removing this layer, a second layer of dissection is initiated to remove as much stromal fibers as possible without compromising the DM. The dissection is continued until at least 95% of the stromal fibers are removed. The edges are dissected with the help of fine Vannas scissors (Figures 10-2D through 10-2G). After completing lamellar dissection of the host bed, the donor tissue is prepared by peeling off the DM-endothelium complex. Donor tissue trephination is done with 0.5 mm oversized trephine. This is then placed over the host bed and sutured with 16 interrupted 10-0 monofilament nylon sutures (Figures 102H and 10-2I). Care should be taken to avoid passage of full-thickness sutures.

A Successful DALK in cases of chemical injury usually results in excellent outcome (Figures 10-3 and 10-4).

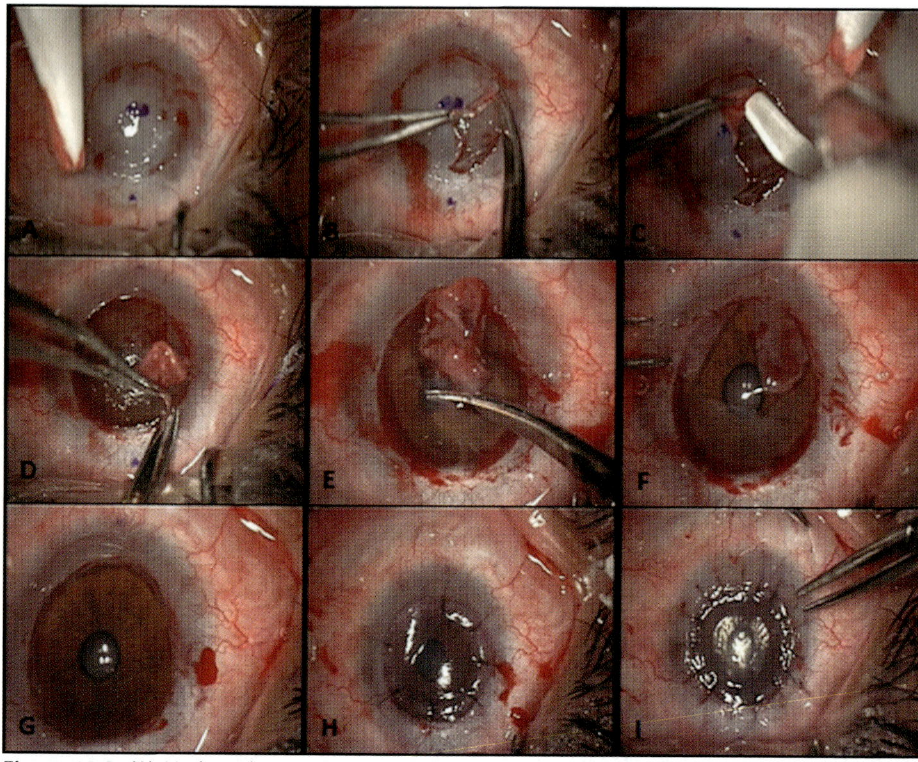

Figure 10-2. (A) Mark on host cornea accentuated by drying with cellulose sponge after partial-thickness corneal trephination. (B-D) Dissection of superficial layer of host cornea with the aid of curved Vannas scissors and crescent blade. (E, F) Dissection of deep stroma by dividing it into 4 quadrants to expose the bare DM. (G) Exposure of bare DM. (H, I) Suturing of the donor corneal button to the host bed.

In cases where, in addition to DALK, extensive symblepharon release has been performed with consequent areas of exposed sclera, an amniotic membrane transplant is usually simultaneously performed.

DALK and Limbal Stem Cell Transplantation

Limbal stem cell deficiency is a major concern when performing keratoplasty in cases of chemical injury as it results in poor healing of the corneal epithelium with persistent epithelial defects, ongoing inflammation increasing the risk of graft rejection and recurrent symblepharon formation. To overcome these problems, it is advisable to stabilize the ocular surface with limbal stem cell transplant prior to keratoplasty. In cases of unilateral chemical injury, an autograft transplant (ie, simple limbal epithelial transplant) is performed, while in cases of bilateral chemical injury either autograft (ie, cultivated limbal epithelial transplant) or allograft transplant (ie, living donor or cadaveric limbal stem cell transplant) is performed.[23-25] Autograft is

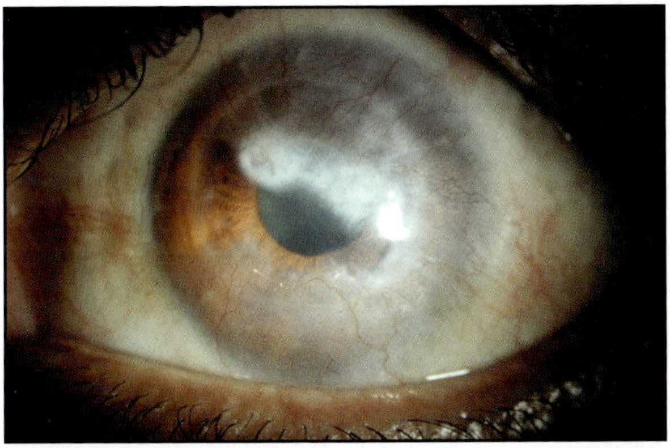

Figure 10-3. A case of chuna particle injury managed with DALK presented with conjunctivalization at 1 month.

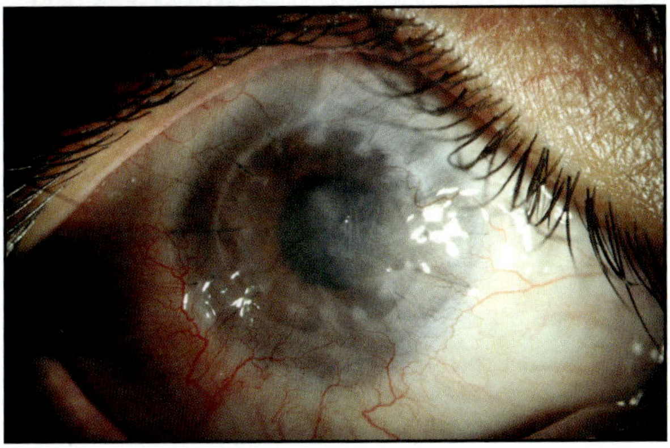

Figure 10-4. A case of chemical injury managed with DALK.

preferred wherever possible as there is no risk of graft rejection and also no need for immunosuppressive medication to prevent the same.[26] One of the major concerns is to decide the time interval between surface stabilization and corneal transplant surgery. A few authors have suggested an interval of 6 months between these 2 procedures.

A few authors have described a technique of DALK with conjunctival limbal autograft performed as a single-stage procedure.[27,28] The rationale behind this concept of single-stage procedure being that keratoplasty performed subsequent to stem cell transplant can itself result in stress to the transplanted stem cells. In this technique a conjunctival limbal autograft is harvested from the normal fellow eye. The graft is then transplanted onto the recipient's superior corneal limbus with 10-0 nylon suture.[27]

Complications

DALK in complex situations understandably has a complication rate higher than when performed for routine cases, like keratoconus.

Intraoperative Complications

Microperforation

The rate of microperforation varies from 9.9 % to 14.2%. In case a microperforation is noted during dissection, an air bubble is injected into the anterior chamber and dissection is continued carefully.[27,29]

Macroperforation

As in any routine case of DALK, large DM tears can occur, and it may be necessary to convert the procedure to a full-thickness keratoplasty.

Postoperative Complications

Epithelial Defect

The mean time for healing of epithelial defect varies between 8 to 14 days, which is longer than that following routine indications for DALK.[29]

Pseudo Anterior Chamber

Formation of pseudo anterior chamber due to collection of fluid between the donor tissue and host bed can occur when a microperforation is missed intraoperatively. Though most cases resolve spontaneously, few cases require pneumopexy for the same.

Graft Edema

Persistent graft edema may occur as a consequence of poor functioning of the host endothelium. It is therefore essential to ensure preoperatively that host endothelium is normal. Preoperative clinical assessment of the endothelium on slit lamp examination is difficult due to the presence of corneal haze. In vivo confocal microscopy can help in this situation to rule out any abnormalities of the host endothelium.[27]

Graft Failure

Graft failure has been reported following graft infection, graft rejection, and poor host endothelial status.

Outcomes

Fogla et al,[27] in a case series of 7 patients, wherein a single-stage DALK with limbal stem cell transplant was performed, reported an average BCVA of 20/50. The ocular surface remained stable throughout the follow-up period (mean duration of follow up: 16.5 ± 5 months). All cases showed remarkable improvement in their ocular symptoms. No complication was noted in the fellow eye as well. Singh et al,[29] in their case series of 9 patients, wherein DALK was performed following simple limbal epithelial transplantation in pediatric cases of unilateral chemical injury, reported an average BCVA of 0.6 ± 0.2 logMAR units. The authors reported an anatomical success rate of 72.72% with a visual success rate of 54.54% only. Amblyopia was considered to be an important limiting factor in this case series.[29]

DALK in Acute Hydrops

The Jacob modification of PD-DALK can be used as a primary management technique for acute hydrops to prevent scarring as described in their report.[30,31] It also provides earlier and faster visual rehabilitation through a single-step surgery. It decreases contact lens dependence and patients may be better able to tolerate spectacles after surgery as this single-staged treatment of acute hydrops gives visual, optical, topographic, biomechanical, and structural improvement in these advanced cases of keratoconus while at the same time avoiding the scarring that is seen after conventional management of acute hydrops. Scar formation after conventional management strategies for acute hydrops can lead to difficult PD-DALK even if the scar is in the periphery, and in case of scarring over the visual axis, can lead to the need for a PK with its attendant lifelong increased risk of graft rejection.

References

1. Maharana PK, Sahay P, Singhal D, Garg I, Titiyal JS, Sharma N. Component corneal surgery: an update. *Indian J Ophthalmol.* 2017;65:658-672.
2. Maharana PK, Agarwal K, Jhanji V, Vajpayee RB. Deep anterior lamellar keratoplasty for keratoconus: a review. *Eye Contact Lens.* 2014;40:382-389.
3. Sharma N, Sachdev R, Jhanji V, Titiyal JS, Vajpayee RB. Therapeutic keratoplasty for microbial keratitis. *Curr Opin Ophthalmol.* 2010;21:293-300.
4. Anshu A, Parthasarathy A, Mehta JS, Htoon HM, Tan DTH. Outcomes of therapeutic deep lamellar keratoplasty and penetrating keratoplasty for advanced infectious keratitis: a comparative study. *Ophthalmology.* 2009;116:615-623.
5. Ti S-E, Scott JA, Janardhanan P, Tan DTH. Therapeutic keratoplasty for advanced suppurative keratitis. *Am J Ophthalmol.* 2007;143:755-762.
6. Parthasarathy A, Tan DT. Deep lamellar keratoplasty for acanthamoeba keratitis. *Cornea.* 2007;26:1021-103.
7. Gao S, Li S, Liu L, Wang Y, Ding H, Li L, Zhong X. Early changes in ocular surface and tear inflammatory mediators after small-incision lenticule extraction and femtosecond laser-assisted laser in situ keratomileusis. *PLoS One.* 2014;9(9):e107370.
8. Sarnicola E, Sarnicola C, Sabatino F, Tosi GM, Perri P, Sarnicola V. Early deep anterior lamellar keratoplasty (DALK) for Acanthamoeba keratitis poorly responsive to medical treatment. *Cornea.* 2016;35:1-5.
9. Wang J, Zhao G, Xie L, Chen M, Zhao J. Therapeutic effect of deep anterior lamellar keratoplasty for active or quiescent herpetic stromal keratitis. *Graefes Arch Clin Exp Ophthalmol.* 2012;250:1187-1194.
10. Ang M, Mehta JS, Mantoo S, Tan D. Deep anterior lamellar keratoplasty to treat microsporidial stromal keratitis. *Cornea.* 2009;28:832-835.
11. Sharma N, Kumar C, Mannan R, Titiyal JS, Vajpayee RB. Surgical technique of deep anterior lamellar keratoplasty in descemetoceles. *Cornea* 2010;29:1448-1451
12. Gao H, Song P, Echegaray JJ, et al. Big bubble deep anterior lamellar keratoplasty for management of deep fungal keratitis. *J Ophthalmol.* 2014;2014:209759.
13. Susiyanti M, Mehta JS, Tan DT. Bilateral deep anterior lamellar keratoplasty for the management of bilateral post-LASIK mycobacterial keratitis. *J Cataract Refract Surg.* 2007;33:1641-1643.
14. Liu X, Zhou Q, Huang X, Liu Z, Bi Y. Clinical evaluation of deep anterior lamellar keratoplasty using glycerol-cryopreserved corneal tissues for refractory herpetic stromal keratitis: an observational study. *Medicine (Baltimore).* 2016;95:e4892.

15. Deshpande S, Banerjee K, Biswas PS, Rouse BT. Herpetic eye disease: immunopathogenesis and therapeutic measures. *Expert Rev Mol Med.* 2004;6:1-14.
16. Shimazaki J, Shimmura S, Ishioka M, Tsubota K. Randomized clinical trial of deep lamellar keratoplasty vs penetrating keratoplasty. *Am J Ophthalmol.* 2002;134:159-165.
17. Sarnicola V, Toro P, Sarnicola C, Sarnicola E, Ruggiero A. Long-term graft survival in deep anterior lamellar keratoplasty. *Cornea.* 2012;31:621-626.
18. Leccisotti A. Air-assisted manual deep anterior lamellar keratoplasty for treatment of herpetic corneal scars. *Cornea.* 2009;28:728-731.
19. Awan MA, Roberts F, Hegarty B, Ramaesh K. The outcome of deep anterior lamellar keratoplasty in herpes simplex virus-related corneal scarring, complications and graft survival. *Br J Ophthalmol.* 2010;94:1300-1303.
20. Sarnicola V, Toro P. Deep anterior lamellar keratoplasty in herpes simplex corneal opacities. *Cornea.* 2010;29:60-64.
21. Dua HS, Miri A, Alomar T, Yeung AM, Said DG. The role of limbal stem cells in corneal epithelial maintenance: testing the dogma. *Ophthalmology.* 2009;116:856-863.
22. Basu S, Mohamed A, Chaurasia S, Sejpal K, Vemuganti GK, Sangwan VS. Clinical outcomes of penetrating keratoplasty after autologous cultivated limbal epithelial transplantation for ocular surface burns. *Am J Ophthalmol.* 2011;152:917-924.
23. Holland EJ. Management of limbal stem cell deficiency: a historical perspective, past, present, and future. *Cornea.* 2015;34(suppl 10):S9-S15.
24. Sharma S, Tandon R, Mohanty S, et al. Culture of corneal limbal epithelial stem cells: experience from benchtop to bedside in a tertiary care hospital in India. *Cornea.* 2011;30(11):1223-1232.
25. Basu S, Sureka SP, Shanbhang SS, Kethiri AR, Singh V, Sangwan VS. Simple limbal epithelial transplantation: long-term clinical outcomes in 125 cases of unilateral chronic ocular surface burns. *Ophthalmology.* 2016;123(5):1000-1010.
26. Dua H, Azura-Blanco A. Autologous limbal transplantation in patients with unilateral corneal stem cell deficiency. *Br J Ophthalmol.* 2000;84(3):273-278.
27. Fogla R, Padmanabhan P. Deep anterior lamellar keratoplasty combined with autologous limbal stem cell transplantation in unilateral severe chemical injury. *Cornea.* 2005;24:421-425.
28. Yao Y-F, Zhang B, Zhou P, Jiang J-K. Autologous limbal grafting combined with deep lamellar keratoplasty in unilateral eye with severe chemical or thermal burn at late stage. *Ophthalmology.* 2002;109:2011-2017.
29. Singh D, Vanathi M, Gupta C, Gupta N, Tandon R. Outcomes of deep anterior lamellar keratoplasty following autologous simple limbal epithelial transplant in pediatric unilateral severe chemical injury. *Indian J Ophthalmol.* 2017;65:217-222.
30. Jacob S, Narasimhan S, Agarwal A, Sambath J, Umamaheshwari G, Saijimol AI. Primary modified predescemetic deep anterior lamellar keratoplasty in acute corneal hydrops. *Cornea.* 2018; 37(10):1328-1333.
31. Jacob S. Primary predescemetic DALK for acute hydrops Soosan Jacob with audio [video]. YouTube. https://www.youtube.com/watch?v=5ZeAXOmVDJw. Published June 14, 2018. Accessed September 27, 2018.

Please see videos on the accompanying website at
www.healio.com/books/DALKvideos

11

Complications After DALK

Claudia Perez-Straziota, MD and Ronald N. Gaster, MD, FACS

Anterior lamellar keratoplasty (ALK) has been proposed as an alternative for patients with corneal disease confined to the anterior aspect of the cornea. It offers the advantage of superior structural integrity compared to penetrating keratoplasty (PK), as well as the absence of endothelial graft rejection, as the host's endothelium is preserved (Figure 11-1). With the introduction of deep anterior lamellar keratoplasty (DALK) and Anwar's big bubble technique for stromal removal, ALK has regained popularity in the area of lamellar keratoplasty. Many of the complications after DALK are somewhat similar to PK; however, there are some complications specifically associated with DALK that will be discussed in this chapter. For the sake of simplicity, the complications have been divided into intra- and postoperative; however, many of the complications that have occurred from surgical technique manifest in the early postoperative period. Prompt diagnosis and management of these complications is of utmost importance to maximize the chance of graft survival.

Intraoperative Complications

Descemet's Perforation

Inadvertent perforation of Descemet's membrane (DM) can occur during stromal dissection, especially in cases of incomplete big bubble formation that requires manual dissection of the stroma[1] (Figures 11-2 and 11-3). DM perforation occurs more frequently in patients with advanced keratoconus who have abnormally thin corneas,

Jacob S, ed. *Mastering DALK: A Video Textbook on Deep Anterior Lamellar Keratoplasty* (pp 127-148).

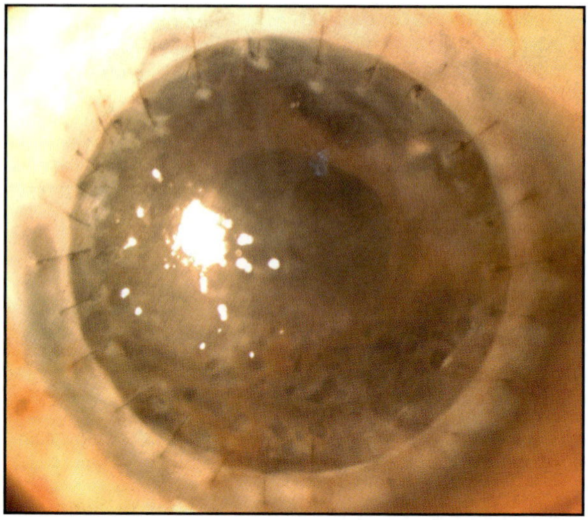

Figure 11-1. Post-PK rejection and graft failure. (Reprinted with permission from Dr. Soosan Jacob, Dr. Agarwal's Eye Hospital, Chennai, India.)

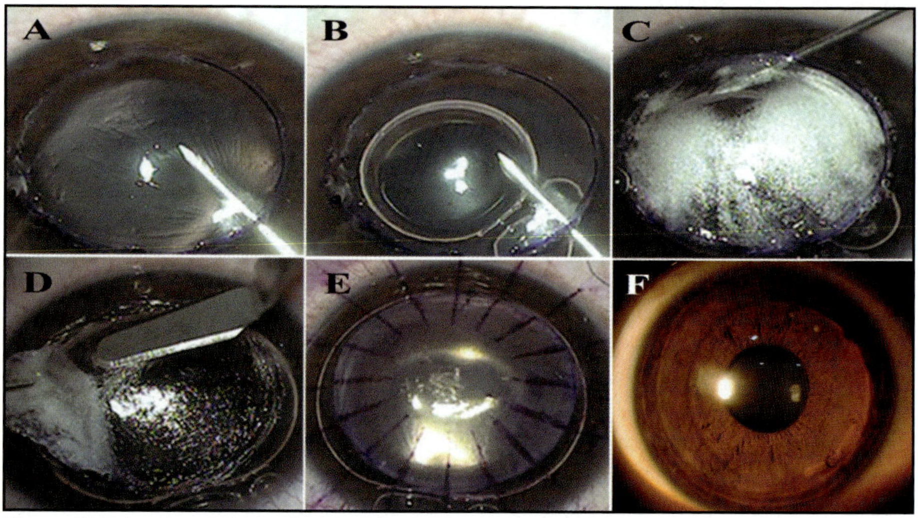

Figure 11-2. Intraoperative perforation during injection. (A) Needle advanced into corneal stroma. (B) Accidental DM perforation leads to bubble entering the anterior chamber. (C-E) Manual dissection pre-Descemetic DALK (PD-DALK) done. (F) Two years postoperation. (Reprinted with permission from Dr. Soosan Jacob, Dr. Agarwal's Eye Hospital, Chennai, India.)

and has been reported to occur in 2% to 12% of cases with experienced surgeons.[1-5] Fortunately, the postoperative prognosis when these perforations are successfully managed does not deviate from the expected prognosis in uncomplicated cases,[6-8] because most of the time the DALK procedure can proceed as planned. Hence the rate of intraoperative conversion to PK after small DM perforations has decreased significantly to 2% with the development of new surgical techniques for stromal removal.[4]

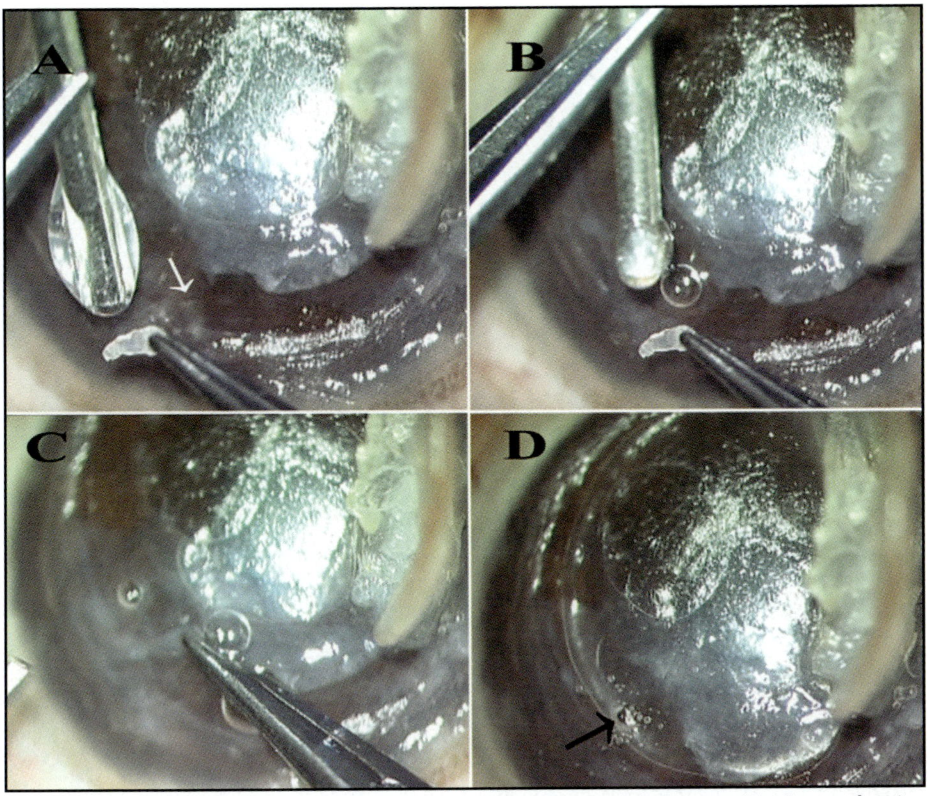

Figure 11-3. Accidental intraoperative perforation during manual dissection. (A) Microperforation seen (white arrow). (B) Fibrin glue applied. (C) Small stromal segment stuck over site of perforation. (D) Perforation sealed (black arrow). (Reprinted with permission from Dr. Soosan Jacob, Dr. Agarwal's Eye Hospital, Chennai, India.)

Depth-adjustable trephines will decrease the risk of perforation during trephination, when the peripheral corneal thickness can be measured prior to surgery (Figure 11-4). A conservative trephine cut to the level of the anterior two-thirds of the cornea is advised to avoid incurring the risk of DM perforation during trephination. Additionally, maintaining a somewhat shallow anterior chamber will not only minimize the risk of perforation but also minimize the size of the perforation should it occur, therefore making it more manageable and increasing the chances of being able to continue with DALK as planned. Perforations can also occur during suture placement; complete Descemet's dissection beyond the area to be grafted provides a peripheral stromal rim that has been dissected off DM and can be used as a holding point for the forceps, providing direct visualization of the stromal thickness to be sutured on the host's side (Figure 11-5).

If a tear in DM is suspected, pressure in the anterior chamber should be lowered to the minimum in order to prevent further extension of the tear. Additionally, once a DM tear has been identified, the approach to dissection of the remaining stroma should be modified accordingly. In perforations less than 2-mm diameter

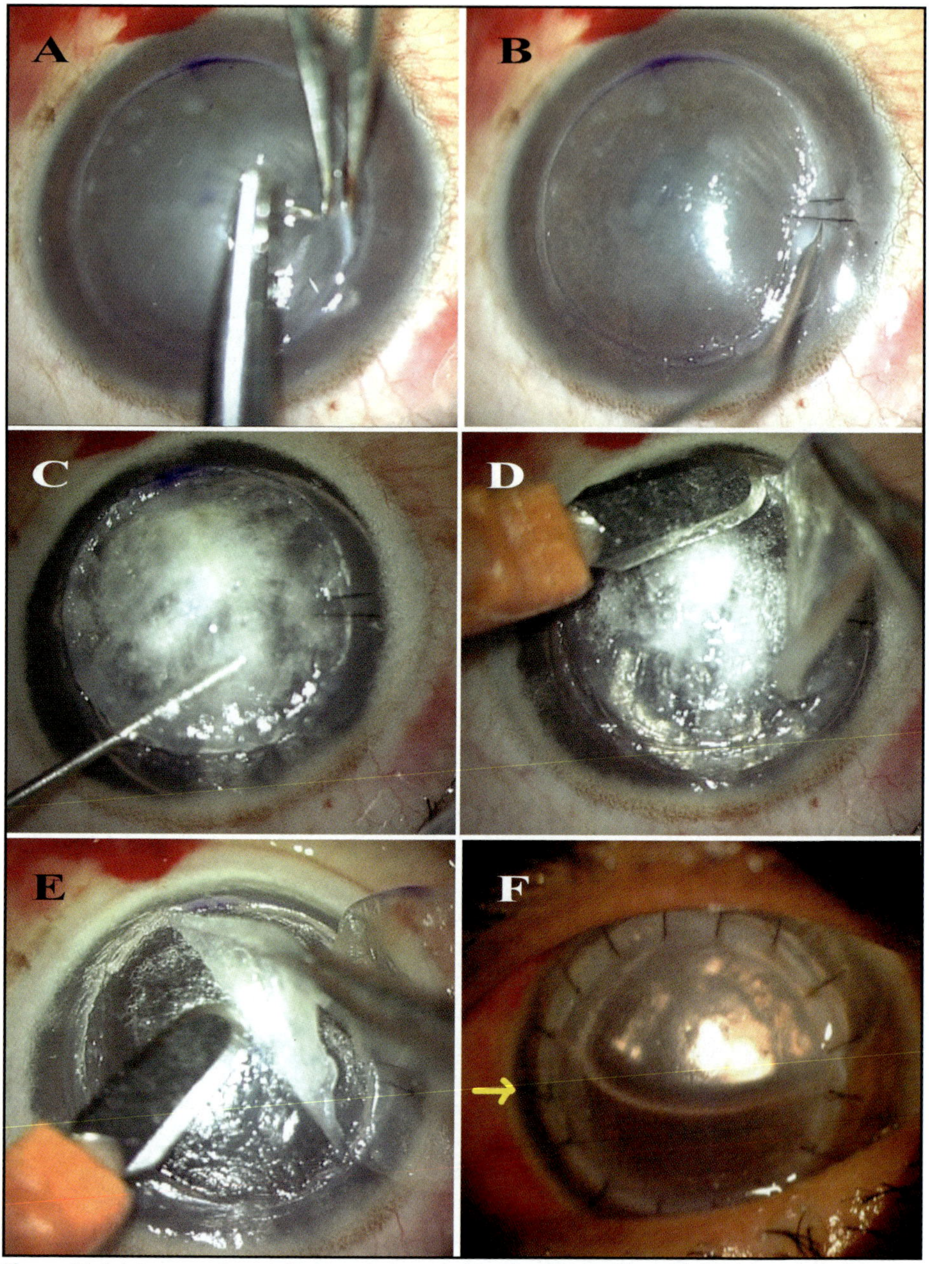

Figure 11-4. Intraoperative perforation during trephination. (A) Accidental full-thickness trephination over 1.5 clock hours. (B) Perforation closed with sutures. (C-E) Manual dissection PD-DALK done. (F) Postoperative day 1 slit lamp picture. Arrow shows site of full-thickness perforation (Reprinted with permission from Dr. Soosan Jacob, Dr. Agarwal's Eye Hospital, Chennai, India.)

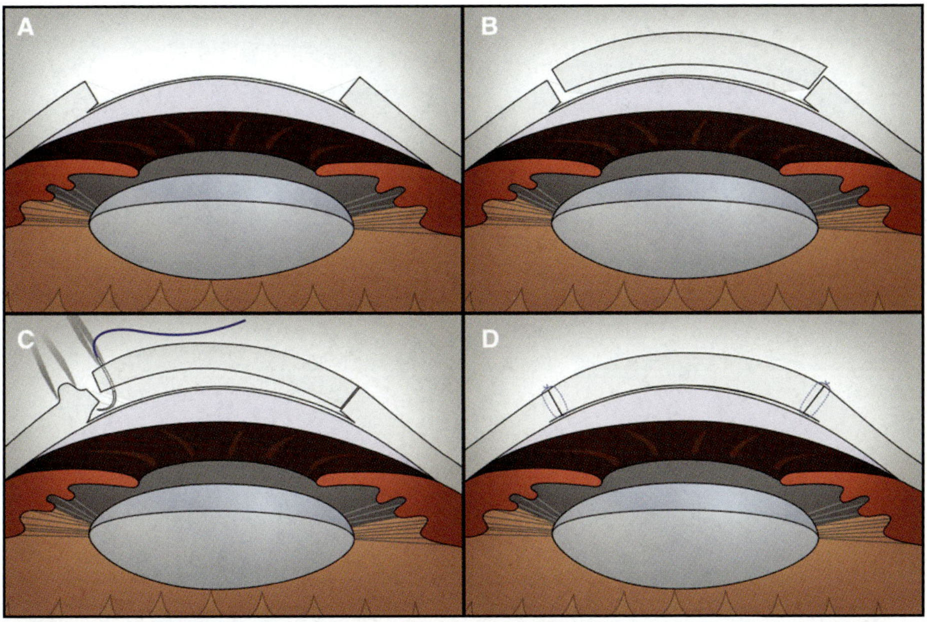

Figure 11-5. (A) Peripheral pocket dissected under host rim. (B) Graft tissue applied. (C, D) Host rim lifted up to pass deep sutures safely without accidentally tearing host DM. (Reprinted with permission from Dr. Soosan Jacob, Dr. Agarwal's Eye Hospital, Chennai, India.)

and located peripherally, the extension of Descemet's dissection can be reduced to the central 5- to 6-mm diameter, as this would still be sufficient for a good visual outcome. However, for larger tears that involve more than 2 or 3 clock hours, conversion to PK is advised in most cases.

Proceeding with DALK when there is a defect in DM should be considered in cases where DALK is going to provide a specific benefit compared to PK, such as highly vascularized corneas, patients with history of infectious keratitis or severe atopia, or patients with severe ocular surface disease. Management options for small tears or perforations include intracameral air injection for tamponade, direct suture of DM to donor stroma when the tear occurs during initial trephination, and in some reports, fibrin glue has been suggested as an alternative for peripheral perforations[9] (Figure 11-6). The most widely use technique, however, is intracameral air tamponade, which will provide support to DM against the donor stroma while endothelial cell migration occurs to heal the tear. This is also proven by the Jacob technique of performing a PD-DALK as a primary procedure for acute hydrops[10,11] (Figure 11-7).

Intra-Descemet's Membrane Air Bubble

DM is ultrastructurally conformed by 2 distinct layers: the anterior, banded zone, which averages 3 μm and varies very little throughout life, and the posterior, non-banded zone, which measures 3 μm for the first 20 years of life and increases thickness thereafter up to 10 to 20 μm at the age of 80. Histological studies of DM have demonstrated that these zones can be easily separated when tangential forces

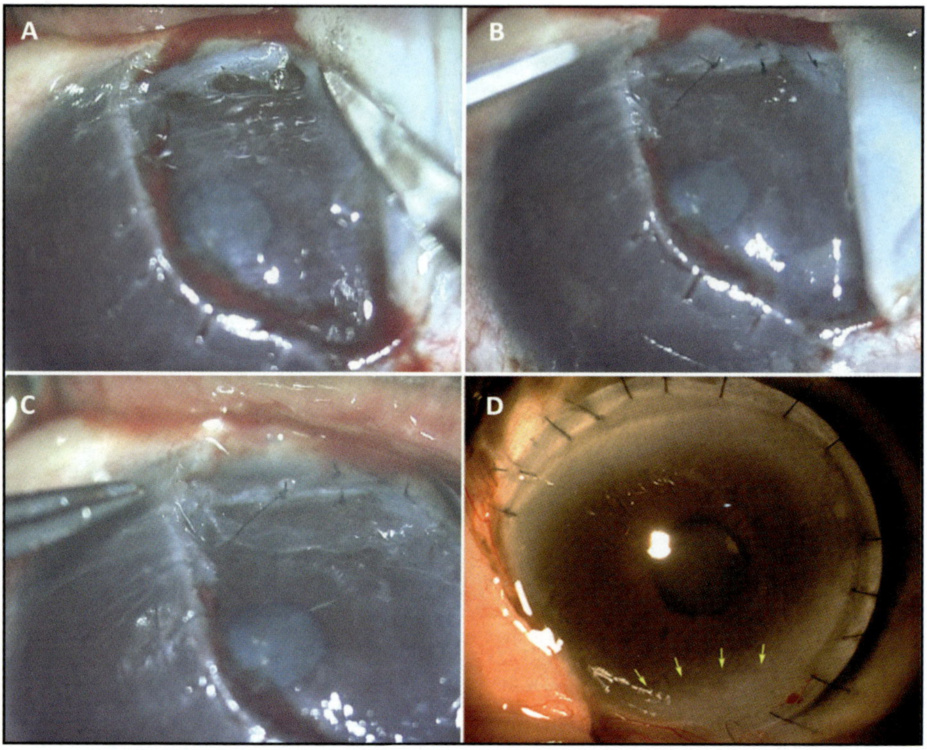

Figure 11-6. (A) Macroperforation seen in PD-DALK. (B) Direct suturing unsuccessful in closing the macroperforation. (C) Small incision lenticule extraction lenticule is stuck with fibrin glue to close the macropeforation. (D) Postoepratively sealed macroperforation, well-formed anterior chamber, and clear graft. (Reprinted with permission from Dr. Soosan Jacob, Dr. Agarwal's Eye Hospital, Chennai, India)

are applied to the anterior stroma.[12,13] In histopathologic specimens evaluated after DALK, Hirano et al[14] observed the attachment of a thin band of DM to the anterior stroma in several cases, proving that the dissection that can appear as to be separating DM from the posterior stroma may actually have occurred through DM separating the 2 distinct bands.

First described by Anwar[15] and Touboul,[16] an intra-Descemet's air bubble can occur when air dissects through DM, separating the anterior and posterior bands. Despite its rare occurrence, cases in which corneal scarring or deep stromal corneal dystrophies, such as corneal macular dystrophy, have increased thickness of the posterior non-banded layer[17] are at increased risk of intra-Descemet's air bubbles.

In comparison with the big bubble, intra-Descemet's air bubbles easily slide under the tip of a fine cannula and are smaller and well-circumscribed. Paracentral bubbles and peripheral bubbles should be displaced as peripherally as possible and very carefully perforated with attention to leave the underlying layer of DM intact. Central bubbles should first be attempted to be displaced peripherally, otherwise the big

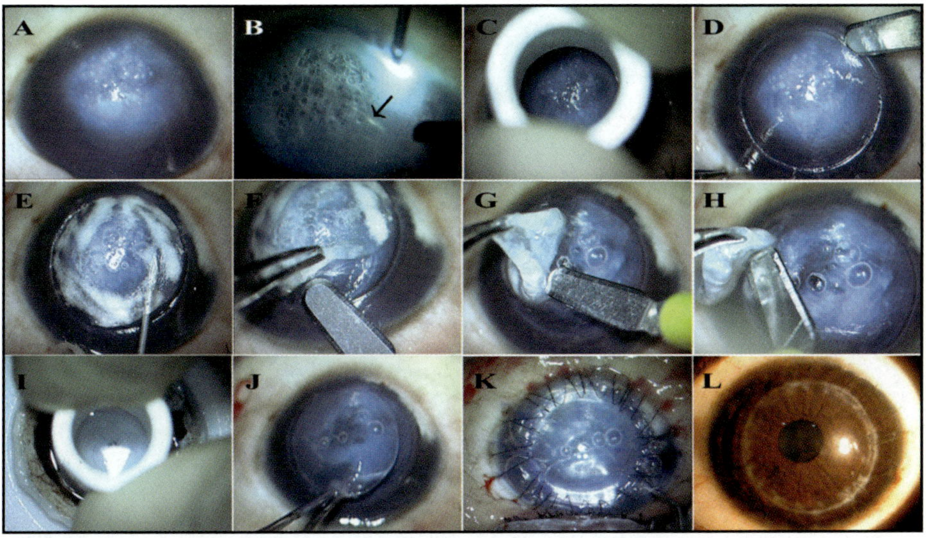

Figure 11-7. Jacob technique for PD-DALK as a primary procedure in acute hydrops. (A) Acute hydrops. (B) Tear in DM seen under the light of endoilluminator (black arrow). (C) Partial-thickness trephination. (D) Groove deepened with crescent blade. (E) Air injected through the bevel up 26-gauge needle to induce emphysema. (F-H) Manual dissection done using the Archilla technique. Deeper layers can be removed with the Melles technique. (I) Donor graft punched. (J, K) Donor graft sutured in place. (L) 13 months postoperative slit lamp picture with 6/12 best-corrected visual acuity. (Reprinted with permission from Dr. Soosan Jacob, Dr. Agarwal's Eye Hospital, Chennai, India.)

bubble must be ruptured along with the intra-Descemet's bubble, also with extreme caution not to perforate the underlying DM. Viscoelastic should be injected into the created space prior to dissection of the remaining stroma in order to protect DM.[17]

Rarely, a PD-DALK may be done over an unrecognized Type 1 big bubble (Figure 11-8), which may then be noticed only in the postoperative period. This generally requires only observation as the big bubble spontaneously gets reabsorbed.

A Type 2 big bubble, if formed, is important to recognize, as these are flimsier and more liable to rupture (Figure 11-9).

Role of Intraoperative Optical Coherence Tomography

Intraoperative microscope-integrated optical coherence tomography can be of use in determining the extent of air penetration into the corneal stroma, depth of trephination,[18] assessment and management of Descemet's detachments,[19] and assessment of iris apposition onto the host's cornea or misdirection of air into the posterior chamber.[20-22] Nevertheless, randomized control studies and standardization of intraoperative protocols are necessary in order to incorporate this technology into the routine surgical procedure.

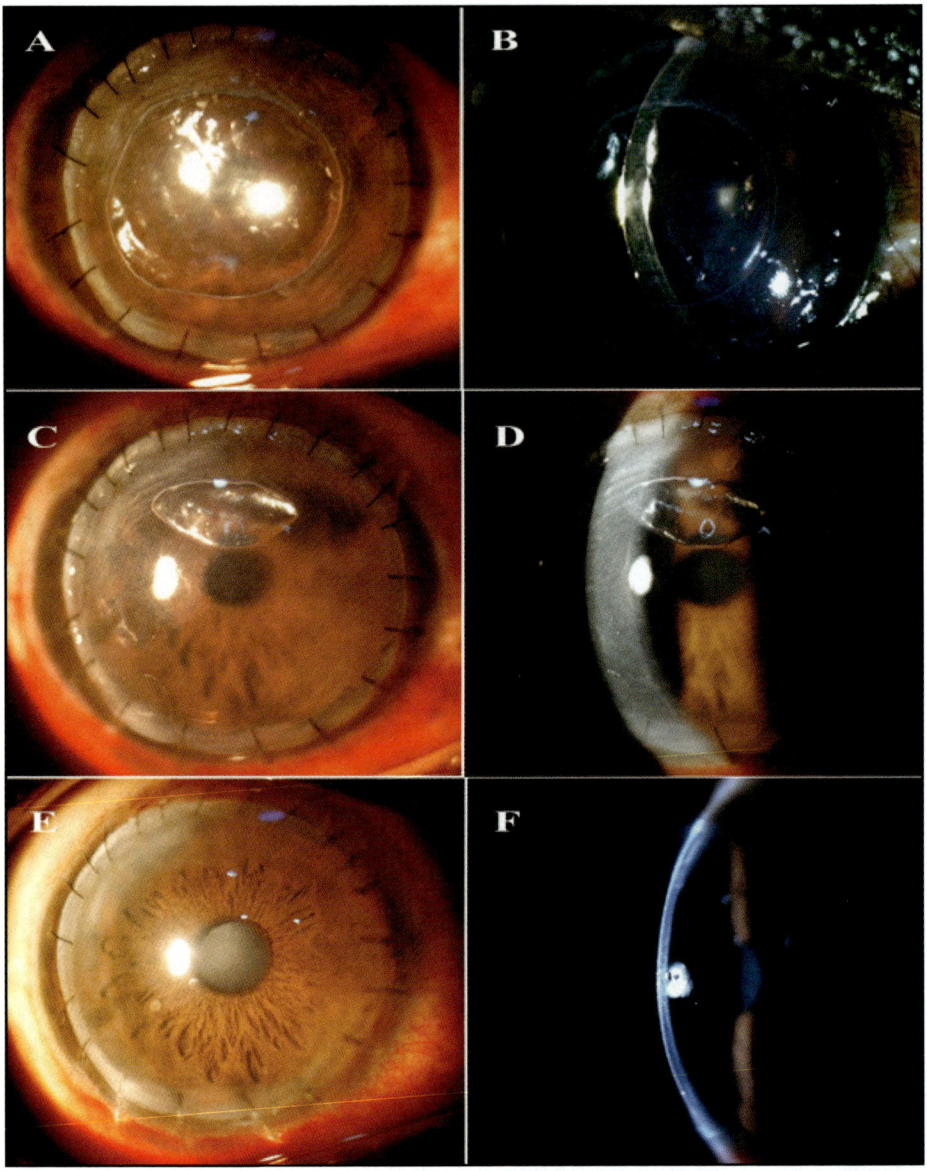

Figure 11-8. (A, B) Day 1 postoperative appearance of PD-DALK. An intact Type 1 big bubble, not identified during surgery, is seen. Surgery was completed as PD-DALK. Graft edema is noticed. (C, D) Absorption of air and decrease in the Type 1 big bubble over next few days. (E, F) Day 10 postoperative appearance. Big bubble fully absorbed, clear graft with resorbed edema is noted. (Reprinted with permission from Preethi S. Naveen, Dr. Agarwal's Eye Hospital, Chennai, India.)

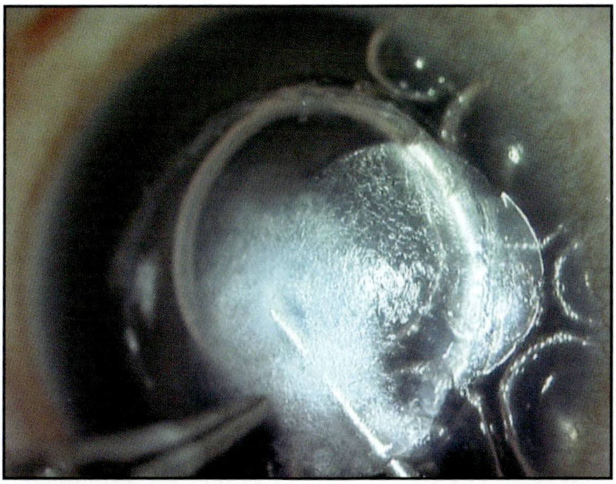

Figure 11-9. Type 2 big bubble obtained during DALK. (Reprinted with permission from Dr. Soosan Jacob, Dr. Agarwal's Eye Hospital, Chennai, India.)

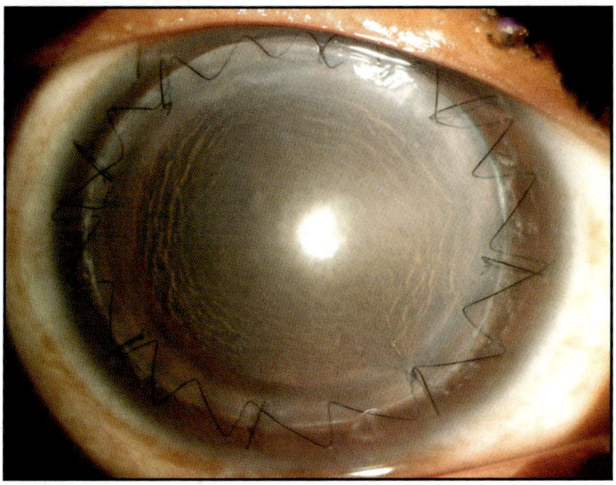

Figure 11-10. Concentric DM folds seen secondary to tight apposition of graft and redundant DM. (Reprinted with permission from Dr. Soosan Jacob, Dr. Agarwal's Eye Hospital, Chennai, India.)

Postoperative Complications

Early Postoperative Complications

Descemet's Membrane Folds

Folds in DM can be seen in early postoperative examinations (Figure 11-10). They occur more frequently in patients with advanced keratoconus,[4] likely from donor-host size mismatch. When located in the visual axis, Descemet's folds can induce glare symptoms or affect visual acuity, likely through inducing higher order aberrations. In contrast, when located peripherally, these folds are usually not visually significant.

Descemet's baring only in the central 5 mm has been proposed as a strategy when performing DALK in patients with advanced keratoconus,[23] in order to leave a peripheral stromal rim that will provide better support to the graft and decrease the chance of postoperative Descemet's folds.

Persistent Epithelial Defects

Early postoperative epithelial defects are very common after keratoplasties in general. In reported studies, 93% of DALK procedures have an epithelial defect on postoperative day 1 that generally heal completely within 3 days. However, persistent epithelial defects, defined as a *non-healing epithelial defects*, lasting more than 7 days, can occur in 2% to 9% after DALK.[24,25] The presence of early epithelial defects is correlated with longer donor preservation-to-surgery times, epithelial sloughing during donor preparation, and quality of the graft in regards to specular microscopy, presence and extent of corneal folds and stromal cloudiness.[24]

Successful management of persistent epithelial defects is important, as they can predispose to the development of microbial keratitis. The placement of a therapeutic soft contact lens with appropriate antimicrobial prophylaxis, amniotic membrane, serum tears, or eventual tarsorrhaphy in recalcitrant cases are all suggested strategies for management. Maintaining topical antibiotic therapy during epithelial healing is of utmost importance to prevent microbial superinfection.

Descemet's Detachment: The Double Anterior Chamber or Pseudo Anterior Chamber

Descemet's detachments, which are usually caused by Descemet's perforations during surgery,[26] occur more frequently when manual stromal dissection becomes necessary due to an incomplete big bubble formation.[1] The double anterior chamber can be easily recognized during early postoperative examinations, delineated by the donor's stroma anteriorly and the host's DM posteriorly. In cases where corneal transparency is compromised and the view to the anterior chamber is poor, visualization of a DM detachment can be challenging. The use of anterior segment optical coherence tomography (ASOCT) can aid visualization of these detachments as well as quantification of their extent (Figure 11-11).

Even though the majority of double anterior chambers are noted in the immediate or early postoperative period, there have also been reported cases of spontaneous Descemet's detachments up to 4 weeks after DALK in patients with advanced keratoconus[26] who had an uneventful early postoperative course. Therefore, careful examination of the anterior chamber should be consistent throughout postoperative visits. A double anterior chamber can also occur due to retained viscoelastic in the donor-host interface, and this can be differentiated from cases due to inadvertent Descemet's rupture by observing the mobility of DM, which is reduced in cases of retained viscoelastic, as well as the degree of corneal edema, which is less in cases of retained viscoelastic.

Although spontaneous resolution of the double anterior chamber has been reported,[3,27-30] these occur mostly in cases where the Descemet's detachment is due to retained viscoelastic. Early intervention with high-frequency topical steroids in small detachments, or insertion of air into the anterior chamber in larger or

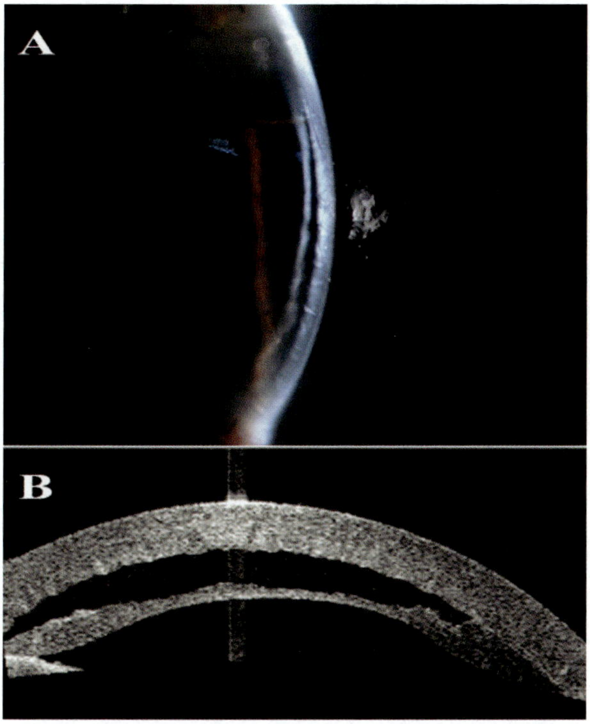

Figure 11-11. (A, B) Double anterior chamber seen on slit lamp examination and ASOCT. (Reprinted with permission from Dr. Soosan Jacob, Dr. Agarwal's Eye Hospital, Chennai, India)

complete detachments, provides faster visual rehabilitation and decreases the risk of fibrosis, which could make management more difficult. In cases where there is no response to early intervention, retained stroma or viscoelastic in the donor-host interface should be suspected, and the interface should be irrigated intraoperatively to remove the retained material.[31] In recalcitrant cases of double anterior chamber where a Descemet's tear had been documented intraoperatively, proceeding to PK as a reintervention is recommended.

Toxic Anterior Segment Syndrome

Despite being mainly an extraocular procedure, toxic anterior segment syndrome has been reported in a case of DALK,[32] most likely due to intraocular penetration with the cannula through the side incision during the instillation of air and/or balanced salt solution into the anterior chamber (Figure 11-12).

Even though endophthalmitis usually presents after the first 24 to 48 hours, and inflammatory findings at this early postoperative period usually point to toxic anterior segment syndrome, there have been reported cases of early onset endophthalmitis, especially from *Staphylococcus* epidermidis and *Bacillus* cereus. Therefore, endophthalmitis should be ruled out prior to initiating treatment with high-dose topical steroids by obtaining aqueous samples for microbiology analysis.

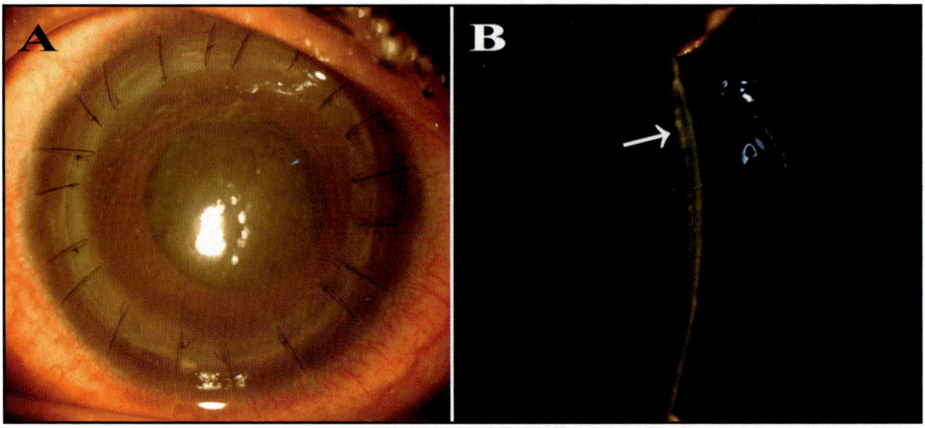

Figure 11-12. (A, B) Inflammatory exudates seen in the graft host interface that resolved with steroids. (Reprinted with permission from Dr. Soosan Jacob, Dr. Agarwal's Eye Hospital, Chennai, India.)

Fixed Dilated Pupil: Urrets-Zavalia Syndrome

The exact etiology of this uncommon complication is still unknown. Iris ischemia and pupillary block related to the injection of air into the anterior chamber have been proposed mechanisms[33,34]; however, it has also occurred after cases that did not require intracameral air injection.[35] An intraoperative peripheral iridectomy or the administration of postoperative mydriatic drops are recommended when air is left in the anterior chamber, to prevent pupillary block and iris apposition onto the peripheral cornea.

Reported as 1.4% in a large case series,[35] Urrets-Zavalia syndrome can result with various degrees of anterior chamber inflammatory reaction and ocular hypertension, but invariably presents with a postoperative fixed dilated pupil with localized posterior synechiae. This change in pupil size is irreversible and can interfere with postoperative visual acuity (Figure 11-13).

Late Postoperative Complications

Interface Opacities

Interface opacities occur most frequently in patients with advanced preoperative ectatic disease (>65 diopters [D] steepest keratometry), and mainly in cases where manual stromal dissection was required due to incomplete big bubble formation.[1] Most of these opacities, such as blood in the interface or interface debris (Figure 11-14), can resolve during the first year of follow up, and only few of them remain visually significant, in which case reintervention with interface flushing or repeat transplantation may be required. In some cases where there is no identifiable etiology, increasing the dose of topical steroid treatment can aid in the control of any inflammatory response that could be generating the opacity. However, close

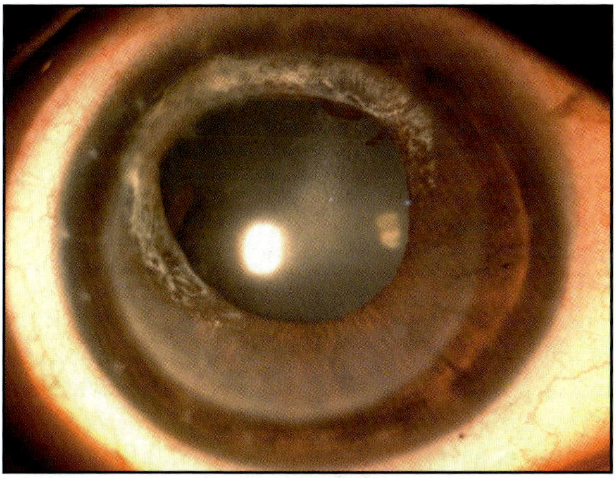

Figure 11-13. Urrets-Zavalia syndrome (fixed, dilated pupil) post-DALK. (Reprinted with permission from Dr. Soosan Jacob, Dr. Agarwal's Eye Hospital, Chennai, India.)

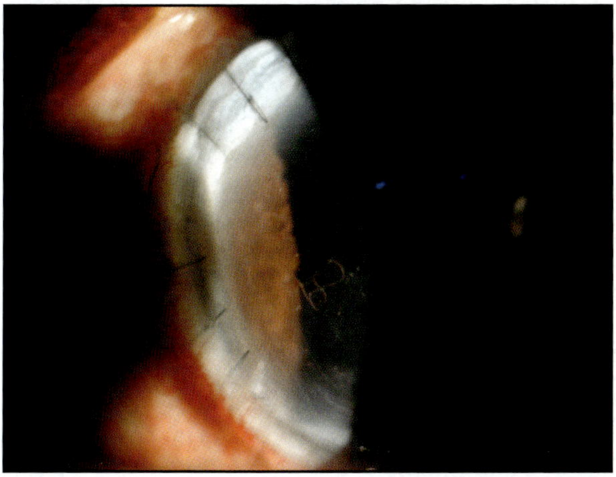

Figure 11-14. Interface debris, pigments, and lint. (Reprinted with permission from Dr. Soosan Jacob, Dr. Agarwal's Eye Hospital, Chennai, India.)

follow-up with confocal microscopy and corneal OCT when necessary, are imperative to rule out microbial interface infection while on high-dose topical steroids.

Infectious Keratitis

The graft-host interface created during DALK offers a virtual space that provides an ideal environment for colonization by micro-organisms that could have gained access intraoperatively or during the immediate postoperative period. The virtual nature of the graft-host interface space challenges the access of antimicrobial agents, making treatment of interface infections rather difficult.

The incidence of infectious keratitis after DALK ranges between 2% and 11%.[36] Identified predisposing risk factors include persistent epithelial defects, use of therapeutic contact lenses, preexisting ocular surface disease, and loose or exposed sutures.[36]

Most cases present within the first 5 postoperative months,[36] and are suture-related or long-term steroid–related infections.[37] Recurrence of herpes simplex virus keratitis has been reported in very few cases[2,38,39] and usually during the first year after surgery[40]; however, the most common etiology of post-DALK infectious keratitis is bacterial.

Common bacterial organisms include coagulase negative *Staphylococcus*, *Corynebacterium*, *Pseudomonas* aeruginosa, *Streptococcus* pneumoniae, and methicillin-resistant *Staphylococcus* aureus.[37,41] Other organisms, such as *Acanthamoeba*,[42] and non-tuberculous *Mycobacteria*[41,43] have also been reported.

Fungal interface keratitis is also a concern after lamellar keratoplasty. The most common fungal organism found after keratoplasty is *Candida* spp,[44] often presenting between 1 and 8 months after the procedure.[44,45] Fungal keratitis is usually seen clinically as multiple whitish-to-yellowish infiltrates at the graft-host interface, and it is important to recognize its clinical appearance despite the lack of inflammatory findings, which is due to the concurrent treatment with topical steroids placating the immune response.[46] If there is doubt about the presence of interface fungal keratitis, treatment with steroids should be discontinued and the patient should be followed closely for the florid manifestation of an infectious process and to obtain adequate cultures. Confocal microscopy can also be an adjuvant in these unclear cases by demonstrating the presence of hyper-reflective 3 and 20 μm granular deposits in the interface.[46]

The role of positive routine donor scleral rim bacterial cultures remains in dispute, because the incidence of bacterial keratitis with positive rim cultures (2%)[47,48] is not significantly different than that with negative cultures (1%).[36,49] In contrast, rim cultures that have resulted positive for fungal infection do increase the probability of fungal infection after corneal transplantation (3%)[50] and show a high correspondence between the cultured organisms in the rim and the causative agent in the recipient's cornea, providing valuable information for treatment adjustment.[49] Therefore, closer postoperative monitoring is recommended when rim cultures yield positive results, especially for fungal contamination; and prompt initiation of treatment according to previously identified susceptibilities is imperative if any clinical findings ensue.

Histopathologic studies of corneas that have undergone PK for recalcitrant microbial infections after DALK have shown the presence of organisms in the deep stroma and in DM.[51] Therefore, the preferred surgical treatment modality in recalcitrant infections is PK instead of repeated DALK, in order to remove all infected tissue. Additionally, a dose of intracameral Amphotericin B can be considered in cases of fungal keratitis in order to eradicate any organisms that may have penetrated the anterior chamber during the procedure.

Secondary lipid keratopathy may be rarely seen following corneal neovascularization after DALK (Figure 11-15). It is, therefore, essential to avoid new blood vessels from growing. New blood vessels may be treated with argon laser photocoagulation, photodynamic therapy, topical steroids, antiangiogenic drugs such as axitinib and bevacizumab topically or as subconjunctival injections, and sometimes direct cautery adjacent to the limbus or fine needle diathermy. Any atopic disease should

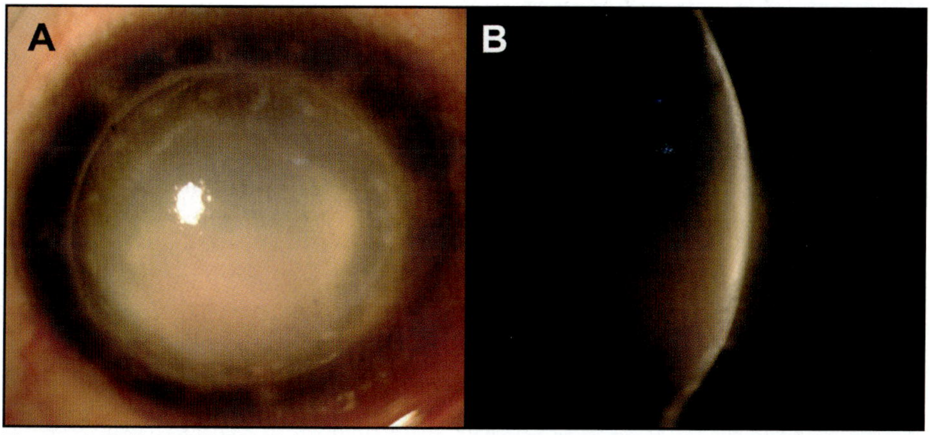

Figure 11-15. (A, B) Diffuse and slit views of lipid keratopathy secondary to corneal neovascularization. (Reprinted with permission from Dr. Soosan Jacob, Dr. Agarwal's Eye Hospital, Chennai, India.)

be aggressively treated, and loose sutures should be promptly removed or replaced as necessary. Lipid keratopathy extending to the visual axis may require a corneal transplantation.

Ocular Hypertension

As topical steroids can be discontinued after the third or fourth postoperative month, the incidence of elevation of intraocular pressure (IOP) after DALK is less common compared to PK. Huang et al[52] reported an incidence of 36.1% of patients, of which 11.4% occurred during the first week and were mostly transient. Their reported cumulative probability during the first year is 30.3%, which remained essentially unchanged throughout the next 5 years. Causes of early elevation in IOP include pupillary block from air in the anterior chamber, reported as 2.5% in a large case series,[2] which can result in Urrets-Zavalia syndrome (ie, irreversible mydriasis) and graft edema in a few cases. Later causes of elevated IOP include steroid response (13.9%),[53] and secondary open angle glaucoma (2.9%).[37] A low percentage of these cases require surgical intervention for IOP management; however, the vast majority are well-controlled with topical treatment.[54] Prevention of IOP elevation after DALK is mostly directed toward minimizing the risk of pupillary block from air in the anterior chamber by ensuring postoperative mydriasis while the air remains in the anterior chamber, or performing an intraoperative peripheral iridectomy. There is no difference in the incidence of ocular hypertension when same-size grafts are compared to oversized grafts.[54]

Endothelial Cell Loss

Up to 5 years after DALK, endothelial cell loss appears to be less compared to PK.[4,55,56] Cell loss has been reported at 8% to 9% at 1 year,[1,2] 10.5% at 2 years, 15.1% at 6 years, and a total of 22.5% at 8 years,[2] with the main proportion occurring during the first 6 months (11%), and then progressively declining in the next 12 and 24

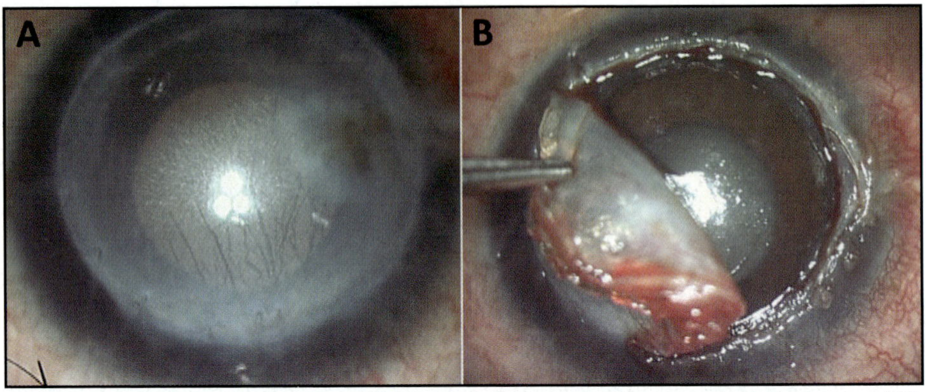

Figure 11-16. (A) Stromal rejection and scarring following extensive neovascularization in DALK. (B) Old DALK graft replaced with new graft. Healthy host endothelium is seen underneath (Reprinted with permission from Dr. Soosan Jacob, Dr. Agarwal's Eye Hospital, Chennai, India.)

months to the physiologic rate of 1% to 2% yearly.[56] Additionally, DALK patients who require subsequent phacoemulsification also appear to be less susceptible to phacoemulsification-related endothelial cell loss compared to PK patients.[55]

Graft Rejection and Failure

DALK is essentially an extraocular procedure. It preserves the host's endothelial cell layer therefore minimizing the chance of endothelial graft rejection, as well as the rate of endothelial cell loss and postoperative glaucoma.[55] However, subepithelial and stromal rejections may still occur. Overall 3-year graft survival has been reported as high as 90% to 98% after DALK[37,57] compared to 94% after PK.[58,59] DALK grafts fail more so due to postoperative complications, such as Descemet's detachment with double anterior chamber, and late infectious keratitis,[60] in comparison to PK, which usually fails due to immunologic graft rejection.[59] The preservation of the corneal endothelium in DALK is why the rate of graft rejection is significantly lower, reported at between 1% and 10%,[2,31,53] compared to PK, reported at 23%.[59] Because the host's endothelium is preserved, endothelial rejections do not occur after DALK; and this is a major advantage, considering that late endothelial graft rejection is believed to be the leading cause of graft failure after PK.[61] Most rejection episodes after DALK originate in the stroma and under the epithelium,[59] and most of them occur within the first year after surgery.[4,31] However, cases of late stromal rejection have been reported up to 46 months after surgery despite complete absence of sutures[62] (Figure 11-16).

Univariate risk analysis of the risk factors for rejection after DALK have shown that young age (< 46 years old), Black race, and trephination cuts (in contrast to laser cuts) all are factors that increase the risk of rejection by 1 year 2.1, 2.7, and 2.7 times, respectively. Additionally, the combination of young age and Black race of the recipient increases the risk by 4.5 times.[63]

Graft rejection after DALK is managed the same way than graft rejection is managed after PK, by increasing the dose of topical steroids to every hour while

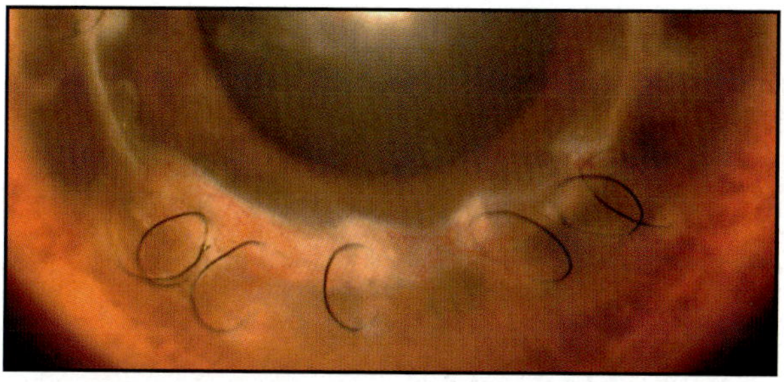

Figure 11-17. Suture-related inflammation and neovascularization in severe atopic disease. (Reprinted with permission from Dr. Soosan Jacob, Dr. Agarwal's Eye Hospital, Chennai, India.)

closely monitoring IOP. All loose or exposed sutures that may be exacerbating the inflammatory response should be removed. The evidence supporting the role of subconjunctival and systemic steroids in the management of graft rejection is not substantial; however, these can be additional measures considered in recalcitrant cases with no contraindications.

Suture-Related Complications

Suture-related complications tend to occur more frequently after DALK compared to PK due to the more superficial placement of sutures. Additionally, suture-related complications are more common in patients with preexisting ocular surface disease, especially atopic disease.[64] Suture abscesses have been reported in up to 18.6% of DALK cases,[53] and should be managed aggressively with suture removal with culture and sensitivities, as well as treatment with broad spectrum antibiotics appropriately adjusted to culture results (Figure 11-17).

In order to prevent and minimize suture-related complications, sutures should be placed meticulously, preferably at a 90% stromal depth in both the recipient and donor corneas with appropriate length and tension. Premature loosening of sutures, especially when they are placed too superficially can occur in up to 26% of cases after DALK,[2,53] posing a risk for infection, suture track vascularization (12.4%),[53] rejection, wound dehiscence, or inflammatory response, resulting in rare instances in postkeratoplasty atopic sclerokeratitis leading to graft melting[65,66] (Figure 11-18). Additionally, spontaneous wound dehiscence after routine complete suture removal has been reported in patients who had any degree of Descemet's compromise, either during surgery or the early postoperative period.[67]

Traumatic Wound Dehiscence

Tensile strength studies performed on cadaveric corneas after PK have demonstrated a rupture pressure of 76 mm Hg for a single continuous suture, 49 mm Hg for 16 interrupted sutures, and 102 mm Hg when femtosecond laser is used to create a top-hat configuration.[68] In contrast, ruptured pressures recorded for cadaveric corneas after DALK are significantly higher, reported between 250 and 300 mm Hg.[69] As some histopathologic reports have shown the possibility of an imperceptible residual stromal layer adhered to Descemet's after big bubble stromal dissection,[70] it is unclear if such stromal remnant contributes to the tensile strength after DALK.

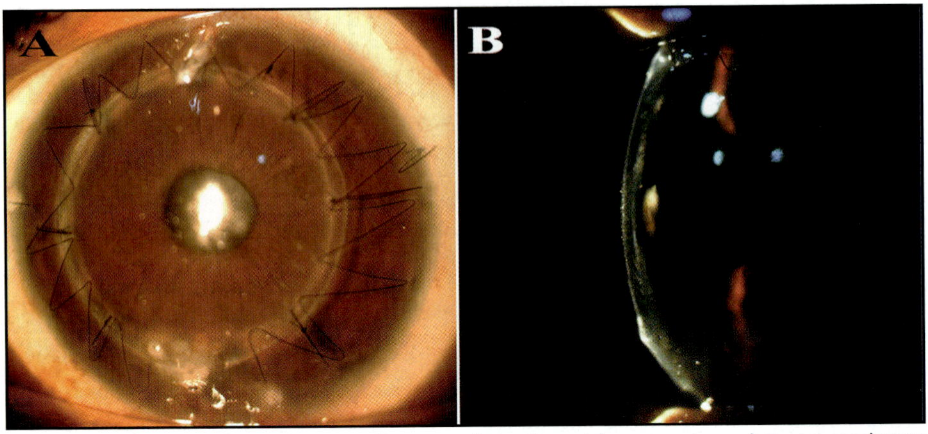

Figure 11-18. (A, B) Graft ectasia, corneal neovascularization, and mucus accumulation secondary to loose sutures. (Reprinted with permission from Dr. Soosan Jacob, Dr. Agarwal's Eye Hospital, Chennai, India.)

It would be reasonable to expect that after DALK, due to preservation of the integrity of DM, most traumatic injuries do not result in wound dehiscence. However, weakness in the graft host junction seems to persist, increasing susceptibility to traumatic globe rupture at the level of this junction. Thus, the site of rupture is invariably the graft-host junction in all reported cases and invariably due to blunt trauma, usually involving 1 or 2 quadrants; and in cases when advanced keratoconus was the indication for surgery, location of rupture is mostly superonasal or superotemporal.

Nevertheless, traumatic wound dehiscence does occur much less frequently after DALK, (0.5% to 3%) compared to PK (2% to 3%).[2,59,71,72] Most cases have been reported to occur within the first year of surgery and in patients whose indication for DALK was advanced keratoconus with abnormally thin corneas.[73] Often, visual acuity after trauma repair does not differ significantly from visual acuity prior to trauma when posterior segment complications do not occur.[73] The corneal endothelium, however, does suffer severe damage after trauma, with reported endothelial cell losses up to 56%.[73]

Conclusion

With the development of surgical techniques, such as DALK with the big bubble technique, that facilitate stromal removal, ALK has reemerged as an alternative for lamellar corneal transplantation that can increase the chance of graft survival in patients at higher risk for endothelial rejection, such as those with preexisting ocular surface inflammatory conditions, as well as provide superior structural integrity compared to PK.

Complications specifically related to DALK compared to PK are mostly related to intraoperative compromise of DM, as well as suture-related complications. Prompt and appropriate management of these complications can minimize the need for reintervention with PK; however, in some instances the safest alternative for the management of both intra- or postoperative complications is to proceed with PK.

References

1. Fontana L, Parente G, Tassinari G. Clinical outcomes after deep anterior lamellar keratoplasty using the big-bubble technique in patients with keratoconus. *Am J Ophthalmol.* 2007;143(1):117-124.
2. Kubaloglu A, Sari ES, Unal M, et al. Long-term results of deep anterior lamellar keratoplasty for the treatment of keratoconus. *Am J Ophthalmol.* 2011;151(5):760-767.
3. Venkatraman A. Spontaneous resolution of double anterior chamber with perforation of Descemet's membrane in deep anterior lamellar keratoplasty. *Oman J Ophthalmol.* 2012;5(2):112-114.
4. Reinhart WJ, Musch DC, Jacobs DS, Lee WB, Kaufman SC, Shtein RM. Deep anterior lamellar keratoplasty as an alternative to penetrating keratoplasty a report by the American Academy of Ophthalmology. *Ophthalmology.* 2011;118(1):209-218.
5. Fogla R, Padmanabhan P. Results of deep lamellar keratoplasty using the big-bubble technique in patients with keratoconus. *Am J Ophthalmol.* 2006;141(2):254-259.
6. Al-Torbak AA, Al-Motowa S, Al-Assiri A, et al. Deep anterior lamellar keratoplasty for keratoconus. *Cornea.* 2006;25(4):408-412.
7. Leccisotti A. Descemet's membrane perforation during deep anterior lamellar keratoplasty: prognosis. *J Cataract Refract Surg.* 2007;33(5):825-829.
8. Khattak A, Nakhli FR, Abdullatif Abouollo HM. Morphometric changes of corneal endothelial cells following intracameral air for micro perforation of the Descemet membrane during big-bubble deep anterior lamellar keratoplasty. *Saudi J Ophthalmol.* 2016;30(2):98-104.
9. Anwar HM, El-Danasoury A, Hashem AN. The use of fibrin glue to seal Descemet membrane microperforations occurring during deep anterior lamellar keratoplasty. *Cornea.* 2012;31(10):1193-1196.
10. Jacob S, Narasimhan S, Agarwal A, Sambath J, Umamaheshwari G, Saijimol AI. Primary modified predescemetic deep anterior lamellar keratoplasty in acute corneal hydrops. *Cornea.* 2018; 37(10):1328-1333.
11. Jacob S. Primary predescemetic DALK for acute hydrops Soosan Jacob with audio [video]. YouTube. https://www.youtube.com/watch?v=5ZeAXOmVDJw. Published June 14, 2018. Accessed September 27, 2018.
12. Murphy C, Alvarado J, Juster R. Prenatal and postnatal growth of the human Descemet's membrane. *Invest Ophthalmol Vis Sci.* 1984;25(12):1402-1415.
13. Sawada H, Konomi H, Hirosawa K. Characterization of the collagen in the hexagonal lattice of Descemet's membrane: its relation to type VIII collagen. *J Cell Biol.* 1990;110(1):219-227.
14. Hirano K, Sugita J, Kobayashi M. Separation of corneal stroma and Descemet's membrane during deep lamellar keratoplasty. *Cornea.* 2002;21(2):196-199.
15. Anwar M, ed. Deep anterior lamellar keratoplasty. In: *Corneal Transplantation.* 2nd ed. New Delhi, India: Jaypee Brothers; 2010.
16. Touboul D, Binder PS, Colin J. Intradescemetic air bubble trapping during deep anterior lamellar keratoplasty. *Cornea.* 2012;31(2):191-193.
17. Sharma N, Swarup R, Bali SJ, Maharana P, Titiyal JS, Vajpayee RB. Management of intra-Descemet membrane air bubble in big-bubble deep anterior lamellar keratoplasty. *Cornea.* 2013;32(9):1193-1195.
18. Pasricha ND, Shieh C, Carrasco-Zevallos OM, et al. Needle depth and big-bubble success in deep anterior lamellar keratoplasty: an ex vivo microscope-integrated OCT study. *Cornea.* 2016;35(11):1471-1477.
19. Sharma N, Aron N, Kakkar P, Titiyal JS. Continuous intraoperative OCT guided management of post-deep anterior lamellar keratoplasty descemet's membrane detachment. *Saudi J Ophthalmol.* 2016;30(2):133-136.

20. Eguchi H, Kusaka S, Arimura-Koike E, et al. Intraoperative optical coherence tomography (RESCAN® 700) for detecting iris incarceration and iridocorneal adhesion during keratoplasty. *Int Ophthalmol.* 2017;37(3):761-765.
21. De Benito-Llopis L, Mehta JS, Angunawela RI, Ang M, Tan DT. Intraoperative anterior segment optical coherence tomography: a novel assessment tool during deep anterior lamellar keratoplasty. *Am J Ophthalmol.* 2014;157(2):334-341.
22. Lim LS, Aung HT, Aung T, Tan DT. Corneal imaging with anterior segment optical coherence tomography for lamellar keratoplasty procedures. *Am J Ophthalmol.* 2008;145(1):81-90.
23. Khakshoor H, Eslampoor A, Rad SS, Vejdani A. Modified deep anterior lamellar keratoplasty for the treatment of advanced keratoconus with steep corneal curvature to help in eliminating the wrinkles in the Descemet's membrane. *Indian J Ophthalmol.* 2014;62(4):392-395.
24. Feizi S, Javadi F, Javadi MA. Graft epithelial defects after deep anterior lamellar keratoplasty. *Cornea.* 2014;33(11):1145-1148.
25. Kocluk Y, Alyamac Sukgen E, Burcu A. Comparison of outcomes in patients who underwent deep anterior lamellar keratoplasty and those converted to penetrating keratoplasty. *Turk J Ophthalmol.* 2017;47(2):63-67.
26. Romano V, Steger B, Kaye SB. Spontaneous Descemet membrane tear after uneventful big-bubble deep anterior lamellar keratoplasty. *Cornea.* 2015;34(4):479-481.
27. Goldich Y, Zadok D, Avni I. Spontaneous resolution of Descemet membrane detachment following big-bubble deep anterior lamellar keratoplasty. *Eur J Ophthalmol.* 2009;19(6):1079-1081.
28. Assia EI, Levkovich-Verbin H, Blumenthal M. Management of Descemet's membrane detachment. *J Cataract Refract Surg.* 1995;21(6):714-717.
29. Minkovitz JB, Schrenk LC, Pepose JS. Spontaneous resolution of an extensive detachment of Descemet's membrane following phacoemulsification. *Arch Ophthalmol.* 1994;112(4):551-552.
30. Mackool RJ, Holtz SJ. Descemet membrane detachment. *Arch Ophthalmol.* 1977;95(3):459-463.
31. Noble BA, Agrawal A, Collins C, Saldana M, Brogden PR, Zuberbuhler B. Deep anterior lamellar keratoplasty (DALK): visual outcome and complications for a heterogeneous group of corneal pathologies. *Cornea.* 2007;26(1):59-64.
32. Sevimli N, Karadag R, Cakici O, Bayramlar H, Okumus S, Sari U. Toxic anterior segment syndrome following deep anterior lamellar keratoplasty. *Arq Bras Oftalmol.* 2016;79(5):330-332.
33. Urrets-Zavalia A, Jr. Fixed, dilated pupil, iris atrophy and secondary glaucoma. *Am J Ophthalmol.* 1963;56:257-265.
34. Tuft SJ, Buckley RJ. Iris ischaemia following penetrating keratoplasty for keratoconus (Urrets-Zavalia syndrome). *Cornea.* 1995;14(6):618-622.
35. Niknam S, Rajabi MT. Fixed dilated pupil (Urrets-Zavalia syndrome) after deep anterior lamellar keratoplasty. *Cornea.* 2009;28(10):1187-1190.
36. Sharma N, Gupta V, Vanathi M, Agarwal T, Vajpayee RB, Satpathy G. Microbial keratitis following lamellar keratoplasty. *Cornea.* 2004;23(5):472-478.
37. Ogawa A, Yamaguchi T, Mitamura H, et al. Aetiology-specific comparison of long-term outcome of deep anterior lamellar keratoplasty for corneal diseases. *Br J Ophthalmol.* 2016;100(9):1176-1182.
38. Leccisotti A. Air-assisted manual deep anterior lamellar keratoplasty for treatment of herpetic corneal scars. *Cornea.* 2009;28(7):728-731.
39. Sarnicola V, Toro P. Deep anterior lamellar keratoplasty in herpes simplex corneal opacities. *Cornea.* 2010;29(1):60-64.
40. Ren Y, Wang H, Zheng Q, et al. Long-term outcomes of deep anterior lamellar keratoplasty treating posterior stroma-implicated herpetic corneal opacities. *Cornea.* 2016;35(3):299-304.
41. Reddy JC, Murthy SI, Vaddavalli PK, et al. Clinical outcomes and risk factors for graft failure after deep anterior lamellar keratoplasty and penetrating keratoplasty for macular corneal dystrophy. *Cornea.* 2015;34(2):171-176.
42. Bi YL, Bock F, Zhou Q, Cursiefen C. Recurrent interface abscess secondary to Acanthamoeba keratitis treated by deep anterior lamellar keratoplasty. *Int J Ophthalmol.* 2012;5(6):774-775.
43. Murthy SI, Jain R, Swarup R, Sangwan VS. Recurrent non-tuberculous mycobacterial keratitis after deep anterior lamellar keratoplasty for keratoconus. *BMJ Case Rep.* 2013;2013: bcr2013200641.

44. Keyhani K, Seedor JA, Shah MK, Terraciano AJ, Ritterband DC. The incidence of fungal keratitis and endophthalmitis following penetrating keratoplasty. *Cornea.* 2005;24(3):288-291.
45. Al-Assiri A, Al-Jastaneiah S, Al-Khalaf A, Al-Fraikh H, Wagoner MD. Late-onset donor-to-host transmission of Candida glabrata following corneal transplantation. *Cornea.* 2006;25(1):123-125.
46. Kanavi MR, Foroutan AR, Kamel MR, Afsar N, Javadi MA. Candida interface keratitis after deep anterior lamellar keratoplasty: clinical, microbiologic, histopathologic, and confocal microscopic reports. *Cornea.* 2007;26(8):913-916.
47. Rehany U, Balut G, Lefler E, Rumelt S. The prevalence and risk factors for donor corneal button contamination and its association with ocular infection after transplantation. *Cornea.* 2004;23(7):649-654.
48. Wiffen SJ, Weston BC, Maguire LJ, Bourne WM. The value of routine donor corneal rim cultures in penetrating keratoplasty. *Arch Ophthalmol.* 1997;115(6):719-724.
49. Wilhelmus KR, Hassan SS. The prognostic role of donor corneoscleral rim cultures in corneal transplantation. *Ophthalmology.* 2007;114(3):440-445.
50. Leveille AS, McMullan FD, Cavanagh HD. Endophthalmitis following penetrating keratoplasty. *Ophthalmology.* 1983;90(1):38-39.
51. Fontana L, Parente G, Di Pede B, Tassinari G. Candida albicans interface infection after deep anterior lamellar keratoplasty. *Cornea.* 2007;26(7):883-885.
52. Huang OS, Mehta JS, Htoon HM, Tan DT, Wong TT. Incidence and risk factors of elevated intraocular pressure following deep anterior lamellar keratoplasty. *Am J Ophthalmol.* 2016;170:153-160.
53. Feizi S, Javadi MA. Factors predicting refractive outcomes after deep anterior lamellar keratoplasty in keratoconus. *Am J Ophthalmol.* 2015;160(4):648-653.
54. Huang T, Ouyang C, Hou C, Wu Q, Hu Y. Outcomes of same-size host and donor trephine in deep anterior lamellar keratoplasty for keratoconus. *Am J Ophthalmol.* 2016;166:8-13.
55. Acar BT, Utine CA, Acar S, Ciftci F. Endothelial cell loss after phacoemulsification in eyes with previous penetrating keratoplasty, previous deep anterior lamellar keratoplasty, or no previous surgery. *J Cataract Refract Surg.* 2011;37(11):2013-2017.
56. Van Dooren BT, Mulder PG, Nieuwendaal CP, Beekhuis WH, Melles GR. Endothelial cell density after deep anterior lamellar keratoplasty (Melles technique). *Am J Ophthalmol.* 2004;137(3):397-400.
57. Sarnicola V, Toro P, Sarnicola C, Sarnicola E, Ruggiero A. Long-term graft survival in deep anterior lamellar keratoplasty. *Cornea.* 2012;31(6):621-626.
58. Jones MN, Armitage WJ, Ayliffe W, et al. Penetrating and deep anterior lamellar keratoplasty for keratoconus: a comparison of graft outcomes in the United Kingdom. *Invest Ophthalmol Vis Sci.* 2009;50(12):5625-5629.
59. Borderie VM, Guilbert E, Touzeau O, Laroche L. Graft rejection and graft failure after anterior lamellar versus penetrating keratoplasty. *Am J Ophthalmol.* 2011;151(6):1024-1029.
60. Borderie VM, Sandali O, Bullet J, Gaujoux T, Touzeau O, Laroche L. Long-term results of deep anterior lamellar versus penetrating keratoplasty. *Ophthalmology.* 2012;119(2):249-255.
61. Olson EA, Tu EY, Basti S. Stromal rejection following deep anterior lamellar keratoplasty: implications for postoperative care. *Cornea.* 2012;31(9):969-973.
62. Roberts HW, Maycock NJ, O'Brart DP. Late stromal rejection in deep anterior lamellar keratoplasty: a case series. *Cornea.* 2016;35(9):1179-1181.
63. Gonzalez A, Feng MT, Lee C, Arbelaez JG, Price FW. Immunologic rejection episodes after deep anterior lamellar keratoplasty: incidence and risk factors. *Cornea.* 2017;36(9):1076-1082.
64. Feizi S, Javadi MA, Javadi F, Jafarinasab MR. Deep anterior lamellar keratoplasty in keratoconic patients with versus without vernal keratoconjunctivitis. *J Ophthalmic Vis Res.* 2015;10(2):112-117.
65. Lyons CJ, Dart JK, Aclimandos WA, Lightman S, Buckley RJ. Sclerokeratitis after keratoplasty in atopy. *Ophthalmology.* 1990;97(6):729-733.
66. Tomita M, Shimmura S, Tsubota K, Shimazaki J. Postkeratoplasty atopic sclerokeratitis in keratoconus patients. *Ophthalmology.* 2008;115(5):851-856.
67. Mannan RMJV, Sharma N, Pruthi A, Vajpajee RB. Spontaneous wound dehiscence after early suture removal after deep anterior lamellar keratoplasty. *Eye & Contact Lens.* 2011;37(2):109-111.

68. Bahar I, Kaiserman I, McAllum P, Rootman D. Femtosecond laser-assisted penetrating keratoplasty: stability evaluation of different wound configurations. *Cornea*. 2008;27(2):209-211.
69. McKee HD, Barua A, Brahma AK, Jhanji V, Carley FM. Rupture pressure of the posterior lamella obtained during big-bubble deep anterior lamellar keratoplasty. *Cornea*. 2012;31(11):1285-1287.
70. Jafarinasab MR, Rahmati-Kamel M, Kanavi MR, Feizi S. Dissection plane in deep anterior lamellar keratoplasty using the big-bubble technique. *Cornea*. 2010;29(4):388-391.
71. Meyer JJ, McGhee CN. Incidence, severity and outcomes of traumatic wound dehiscence following penetrating and deep anterior lamellar keratoplasty. *Br J Ophthalmol*. 2016;100(10):1412-1415.
72. Kawashima M, Kawakita T, Shimmura S, Tsubota K, Shimazaki J. Characteristics of traumatic globe rupture after keratoplasty. *Ophthalmology*. 2009;116(11):2072-2076.
73. Sari ES, Koytak A, Kubaloglu A, et al. Traumatic wound dehiscence after deep anterior lamellar keratoplasty. *Am J Ophthalmol*. 2013;156(4):767-772.

Please see videos on the accompanying website at
www.healio.com/books/DALKvideos

12

Interface Tattooing With Fibrin Glue–Assisted Superficial Anterior Lamellar Keratoplasty Using Small Incision Lenticule Extraction Lenticule for Limbal Dermoids

Soosan Jacob, MS, FRCS, DNB, MNAMS and Smita Narasimhan, MBBS

Limbal dermoid is a sporadically occurring congenital tumor that straddles the limbus and is generally found in the inferotemporal quadrant.[1] It is a choristoma, having a keratinized surface with hair follicles seen on the surface. They are classified as Grade 1, which is superficial and measures less than 5 mm; Grade 2, which is larger and also deeper and extends to the Descemet's membrane; and Grade 3, where the entire anterior segment is involved. These can be cosmetically disfiguring, may cause foreign body sensation, astigmatism, lipid infiltration on the cornea, dellen formation, inability to close the lids completely, or, rarely, completely obstruct the visual axis. They may also be associated with other syndromes, such as the Goldenhar syndrome, Duane retraction syndrome, and SCALP (sebaceous nevus syndrome, central nervous system malformations, aplasia cutis congenita, limbal dermoid, pigmented nevus with neurocutaneous melanosis) syndrome.

Limbal dermoids may be observed without necessarily having to be removed, however, because it can be cosmetically disfiguring, many patients/parents of affected children do opt for surgery. If surgery is decided on, various options have been described in the past.[2-5] These include superficial sclerokeratectomy, deep excision with lamellar keratoplasty, amniotic membrane grafting, and full-thickness excision with penetrating sclerokeratoplasty.[1,6-14]

The author (SJ) has described a technique for Type 1 limbal dermoids where a donor lenticule extracted from a small incision lenticule extraction (SMILE) surgery

Jacob S, ed. *Mastering DALK: A Video Textbook on Deep Anterior Lamellar Keratoplasty* (pp 149-156).

for correction of myopia is used for corneal resurfacing after lamellar excision of the dermoid.[15] Interface tattoo is also used to enhance the cosmetic outcome.

Technique

A 26-gauge needle is used to inject balanced salt solution (BSS) under the conjunctiva adjacent to the dermoid. The ballooned free conjunctiva is then dissected off the surface of the dermoid up to the extent possible. An inked trephine is used to mark a shallow groove around the corneal part of the limbal dermoid and this is then deepened with a crescent blade. The dermoid tissue is then dissected in a lamellar plane minimally below the level of the adjacent normal cornea. Dissection is carried onto the scleral surface and the limbal dermoid is thus removed. Any bleeding vessels on the scleral surface are cauterized and the limbal outline contiguous with the adjacent cornea is marked with a fine-tipped marker pen. The circular outline marked is again verified under natural room light illumination with the microscope light turned off, and once confirmed to be contiguous with the darker appearance of the iris seen through adjacent cornea, tattoo pigment (Appasamy Associates) is applied carefully on a dry bed within the circular marked outline of the excised corneal portion of the limbal dermoid. Care is taken to not allow the pigment to spread anywhere outside the marked outline. Circularity and cosmesis is again assessed under room light illumination. A donor SMILE lenticule harvested from a suitably screened refractive candidate (negative for anti-HIV-1 and anti-HIV-2, Hepatitis B surface antigen, anti–Hepatitis C virus, and venereal disease research laboratory test) is then applied to the bed using minimal fibrin glue. Any excess lenticule lying outside the limbus can be trimmed and the conjunctiva is finally stuck into position using fibrin glue. Amniotic membrane may be used to cover any large area of deficient conjunctiva (Figure 12-1).

Advantages

Current techniques for excision have many disadvantages. They may leave a bluish-white scar seen in 50% of cases, which is more markedly visible in dark-colored eyes. Sutured apposition of full-thickness or lamellar grafts can lead to suture-induced astigmatism. Suture bites close to the visual axis cause scars in the line of vision and irregular astigmatism. Scleral outlines of thicker grafts are often visible through overlying conjunctiva, even under room illumination, giving a poor cosmetic outcome.

Our technique has the advantage of using the SMILE lenticule as a thin lamellar graft for superficial corneal resurfacing. SMILE lenticules have already been used in the past for treatment of presbyopia (PrEsbyopic Allogeneic Refractive Lenticule [PEARL], a technique described by one of the authors [SJ]),[16] hyperopia, keratoconus, and other applications with proven safety and efficacy (Figure 12-2).[17-21]

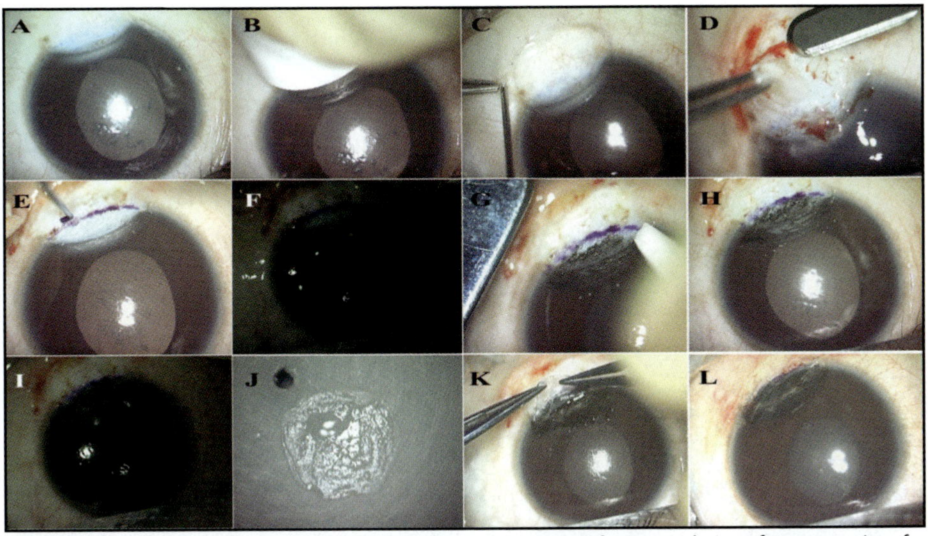

Figure 12-1. SMILE lenticule–assisted sutureless corneal resurfacing with interface tattooing for limbal dermoid. (A) Limbal dermoid—intraoperative view. (B) A circular trephine gently marks the anterior border for excision. (C) Conjunctiva is ballooned in the area of limbal dermoid by injecting BSS. (D) Conjunctiva is cut around the keratinized area and free conjunctiva dissected off underlying dermoid. Limbal dermoid is excised at a lamellar plane minimally below plane of surrounding normal cornea. Dermoid tissue extending over sclera is dissected flush with normal sclera. Bleeding points are cauterized. (E) Circular margin of tattooing is marked with a fine-tipped marker pen. (F) Circularity and cosmesis are assessed in natural viewing conditions with microscope light turned off. (G, H) Corneal tattoo powder is applied on a dry bed carefully following the circular shape marked near the limbus. (I) Circularity and cosmesis are again assessed in natural viewing conditions with microscope light turned off. (J) Donor SMILE lenticule. (K) SMILE lenticule is spread out and stuck with minimal amount of fibrin glue; (L) conjunctiva is stuck using fibrin glue.

Use of the thin, uniform, and regular SMILE lenticule in our technique allows a smooth anterior corneal surface with good postoperative comfort. Fibrin glue allows easy and good apposition of the graft to the underlying cornea, while avoiding disadvantages related to sutures, such as astigmatism, scarring, and loosening of sutures (Figure 12-3). The tattoo applied in the interface gives excellent cosmetic outcome and prevents the white appearance of the residual dermoid tissue from being seen through. The thin nature of the lenticule allows the pigment to be seen through even a mildly hazy graft. The thin SMILE lenticule is also not visible over the scleral surface unlike thicker grafts where the scleral outline is often seen through overlying conjunctiva. Tattoo pigments of different colors may be chosen according to iris color.[22] Application of tattoo in the interface as opposed to surface tattooing gives long-term effect and lasting cosmetic outcomes.

Avoiding deep dissection prevents complications such as intraoperative perforation, postoperative thinned out residual host cornea, limbus and sclera, graft ectasia, and induced astigmatism. Superficial dissection gives superior tectonic stability and, therefore, also better visual acuity. As the SMILE lenticule comes pre-prepared, it allows quick and easy surgery and avoids time spent in deeper dissection, as well as preparation of a graft.

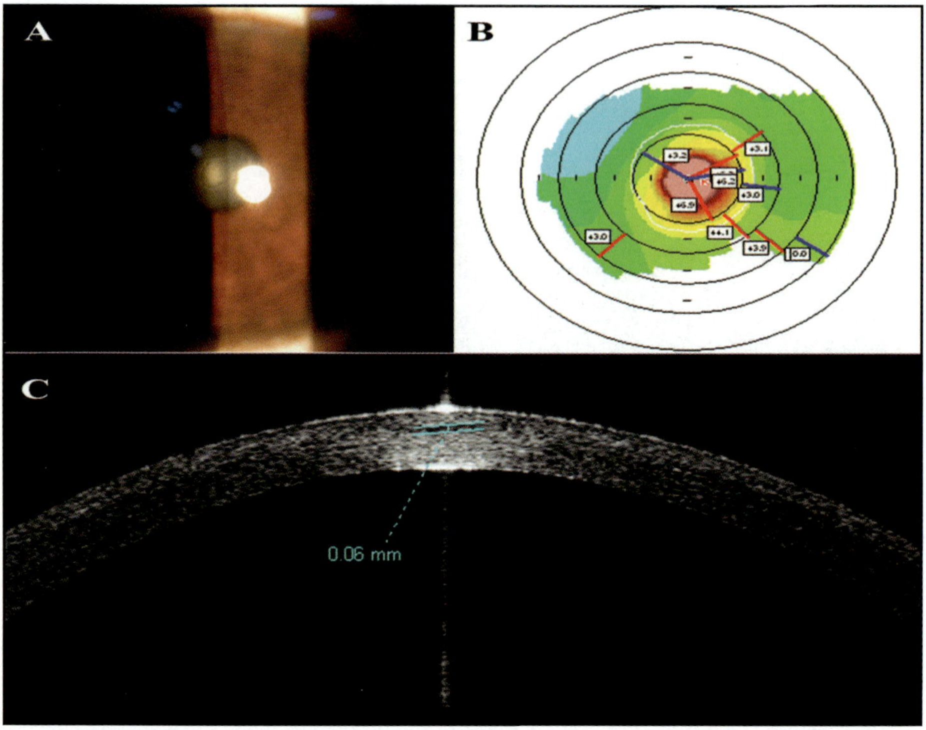

Figure 12-2. PEARL. (A) Slit lamp appearance of PEARL lenticule. (B) Topography of PEARL lenticule showing central hyperprolateness. (C) Anterior segment optical coherence tomography (ASOCT) showing PEARL lenticule within a femtosecond-dissected pocket in the presbyopic patient's eye.

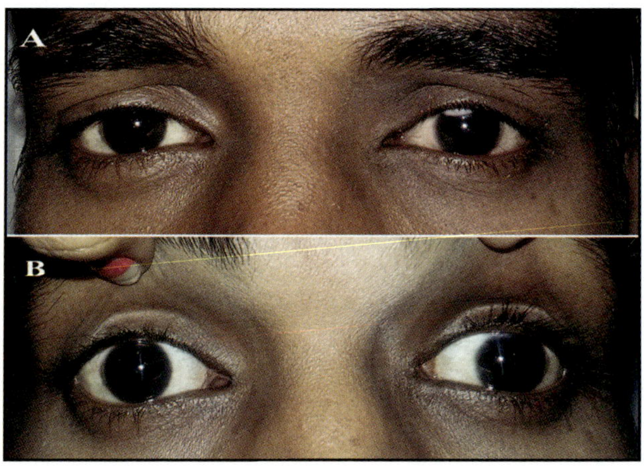

Figure 12-3. (A, B) Pre- and postoperative appearance of sutureless SMILE lenticule–assisted corneal resurfacing with interface tattooing for limbal dermoid excision (superior dermoid—left eye).

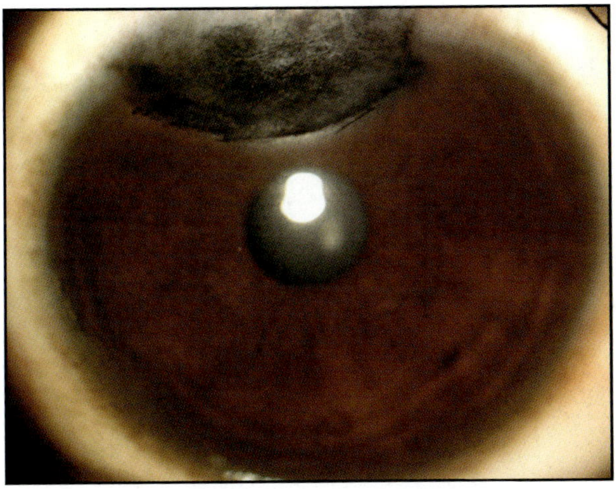

Figure 12-4. Postoperative slit lamp appearance showing a smooth surface, interface tattooing, and a quiet eye.

Disadvantages

The availability of a SMILE lenticule may restrict widespread usage and restrict this technique to centers where SMILE surgery is performed. However, in the future, eye bank involvement for preservation and supply of SMILE lenticules can be the solution. An alternate but similar technique using a microkeratome-created flap of 100 µm or an 80 µm femtosecond LASIK flap on a donor corneoscleral rim has been routinely performed by the author (SJ) in the past with similar good results, and this technique may instead be used in centers without access to SMILE lenticule.

Conclusion

This technique offers advantages of ease, safety, and good cosmesis together with a stable refractive and tectonic outcome. It also decreases the risk of complications such as intraoperative perforation, postoperative limbal ectasia, and visible corneal scarring (Figures 12-4 to 12-6).

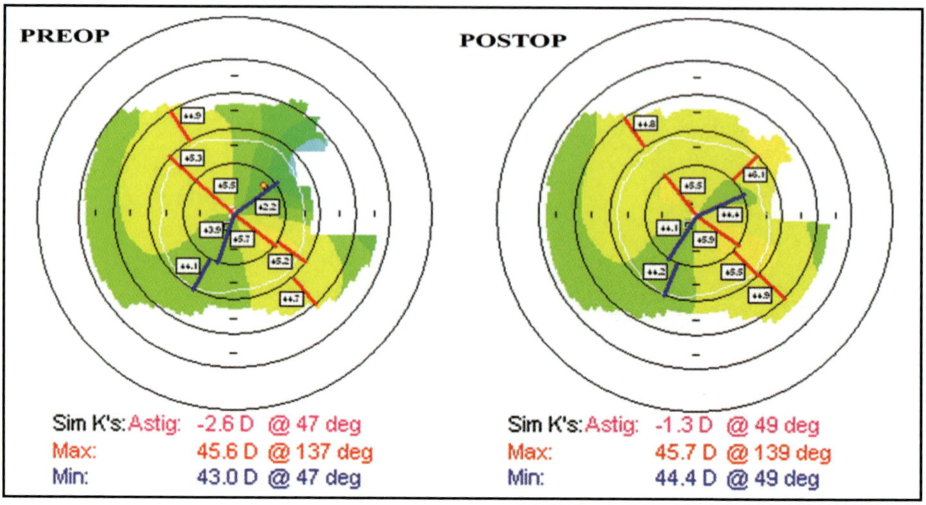

Figure 12-5. Postoperative improvement in corneal astigmatism seen on corneal topography.

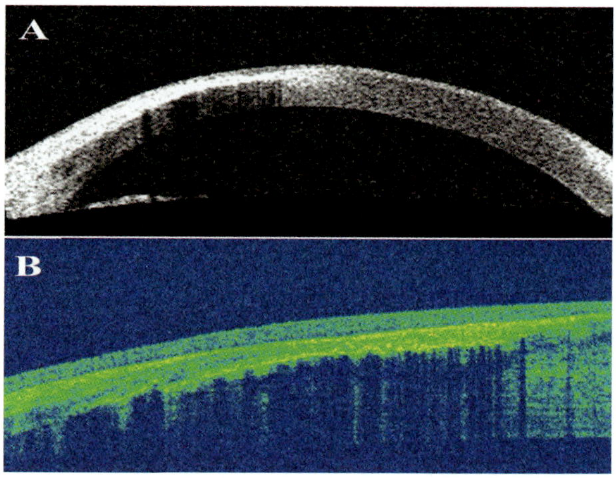

Figure 12-6. (A) ASOCT showing on the left side well-placed and apposed lenticule with interface tattoo and overlying normal epithelium; (B) Fourier domain optical coherence tomography confirming the same.

References

1. Mansour AM, Barber JC, Reinecke RD, et al. Ocular choristomas. *Surv Ophthalmol.* 1989;33:339-358
2. Lang SJ, Böhringer D, Reinhard T. Surgical management of corneal limbal dermoids: retrospective study of different techniques and use of Mitomycin C. *Eye.* 2014;28:857-862
3. Matsuo T. Clinical decision upon resection or observation of ocular surface dermoid lesions with the visual axis unaffected in pediatric patients. *Springerplus.* 2015;4:534.
4. Mohan M, Mukherjee G, Panda A. Clinical evaluation and surgical intervention of limbal dermoid. *Indian J Ophthalmol.* 1981;29:69-73.
5. Panton RW, Sugar J. Excision of limbal dermoids. *Ophthalmic Surg.* 1991;22:85-89.
6. Mohan M, Mukherjee G, Panda A. Clinical evaluation and surgical intervention of limbal dermoid. *Indian J Ophthalmol.* 1981;29:69-73.
7. Panton RW, Sugar J. Excision of limbal dermoids. *Ophthalmic Surg.* 1991;22:85-89.
8. Watts P, Michaeli-Cohen A, Abdolell M, et al. Outcome of lamellar keratoplasty for limbal dermoids in children. *J AAPOS.* 2002;6:209-215.
9. Scott JA, Tan DT. Therapeutic lamellar keratoplasty for limbal dermoids. *Ophthalmology.* 2001;108:1858-1867.
10. Wu KI, Chu H-S, Pai AS, Hou YC, Lin SY, Chen WL, Hu FR. Surgical management of limbal dermoids using anterior corneal buttons from Descemet stripping automated endothelial keratoplasty donor tissue as patch grafts. *Cornea.* 2017;36(1):64-67.
11. Lazzaro DR, Coe R. Repair of limbal dermoid with excision and placement of a circumlimbal pericardial graft. *Eye Contact Lens.* 2010;36:228-229.
12. Pirouzian A. Management of pediatric corneal limbal dermoids. *Clin Ophthalmol.* 2013;7:607-614.
13. Pirouzian A, Holz H, Merrill K, et al. Surgical management of pediatric limbal dermoids with sutureless amniotic membrane transplantation and augmentation. *J Pediatr Ophthalmol Strabismus.* 2012;49:114-119.
14. Zhou AX, Ambati BK. Sutureless lamellar corneoscleral patch graft with fibrin sealant for limbal dermoid removal. *J Pediatr Ophthalmol Strabismus.* 2016;53:E22-E25.
15. Jacob S, Narasimhan S, Agarwal A, Agarwal A, Ai S. Combined interface tattooing and fibrin glue-assisted sutureless corneal resurfacing with donor lenticule obtained from small-incision lenticule extraction for limbal dermoid. *J Cataract Refract Surg.* 2017;43(11):1371-1375.
16. Jacob S, Kumar DA, Agarwal A, et al. Preliminary evidence of successful near vision enhancement with a new technique: presbyopic allogenic refractive lenticule (PEARL) corneal inlay using a SMILE lenticule. *J Refract Surg.* 2017;33(4):224-229.
17. Pradhan KR, Reinstein DZ, Carp GI, et al. Femtosecond laser-assisted keyhole endokeratophakia: correction of hyperopia by implantation of an allogeneic lenticule obtained by SMILE from a myopic donor. *J Refract Surg.* 2013;29(11):777-782.
18. Sun L, Yao P, Li M, et al. The safety and predictability of implanting autologous lenticule obtained by SMILE for hyperopia. *J Refract Surg.* 2015;31(6):374-379.
19. Ganesh S, Brar S, Rao PA. Cryopreservation of extracted corneal lenticules after small incision lenticule extraction for potential use in human subjects. *Cornea.* 2014;33(12):1355-1362.

20. Ganesh S, Brar S. Femtosecond intrastromal lenticular implantation combined with accelerated collagen cross-linking for the treatment of keratoconus-initial clinical result in 6 eyes. *Cornea*. 2015;34(10):1331-139.
21. Bhandari V, Ganesh S, Brar S, Pandey R. Application of the SMILE-derived glued lenticule patch graft in microperforations and partial thickness corneal defects. *Cornea*. 2016;35(3):408-412.
22. Amesty MA, Rodriguez AE, Hernández E, et al. Tolerance of micronized mineral pigments for intrastromal keratopigmentation: a histopathology and immunopathology experimental study. *Cornea*. 2016;35(9):1199-1205.

Please see videos on the accompanying website at
www.healio.com/books/DALKvideos

13

Corneal Allogenic Intrastromal Ring Segments
An Alternative to DALK in Certain Situations

Soosan Jacob, MS, FRCS, DNB, MNAMS

Intrastromal corneal ring segments (ICRS) have been used in the past to treat keratoconus and other ectatic disorders. It is a reversible procedure that flattens the central corneal curvature while leaving the central visual axis of the cornea unaltered. The segments have an arc shortening effect and bring about a regularization in corneal topography; however, in the past, these have been made of synthetic material and have been reported to have up to a 35% complication rate[1] associated with implantation of synthetic substance within the cornea, such as corneal haze, channel deposits, corneal neovascularization, and chronic pain, as well as more serious complications, such as extrusion, erosion, migration, and infectious keratitis.

Corneal allogenic intrastromal ring segments (CAIRS) is a new procedure that was devised by the author and is similar to Intacs (Addition Technology Inc), Kerarings (Mediphacos Inc) but with the distinct advantage of using allogenic tissue[2,3] (Figure 13-1).

Indications

Keratoconus, pellucid marginal degeneration, other causes of corneal ectasias, and irregular corneas are indications for CAIRS implantation. They are indicated in patients with mild to moderately severe disease and unsatisfactory vision with glasses. A clear cornea over the visual axis is a prerequisite.

Jacob S, ed. *Mastering DALK: A Video Textbook on Deep Anterior Lamellar Keratoplasty* (pp 157-166).

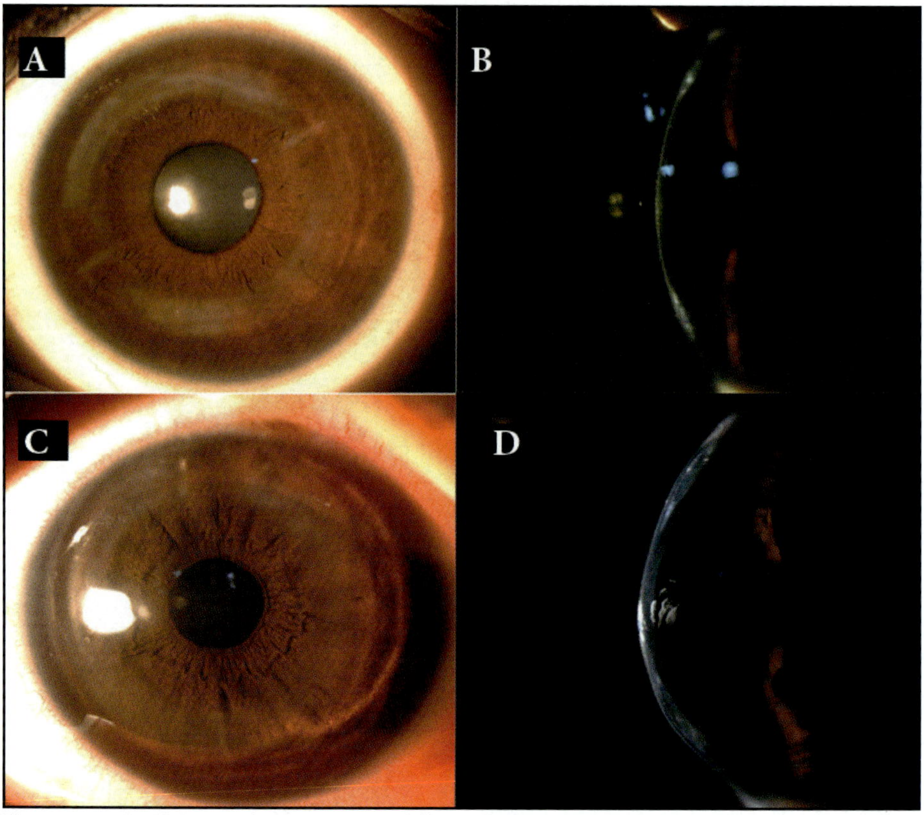

Figure 13-1. (A, B) Pre- and postoperative diffuse and slit beam images of double segment CAIRS. (C, D) Pre- and postoperative diffuse and slit beam images of single segment 340° CAIRS.

Mechanism of Action

CAIRS produces a flattening and regularization of the corneal topography and, therefore, decreases irregular astigmatism, reduces corneal steepening, and improves uncorrected visual acuity (UCVA) and best-corrected visual acuity (BCVA) while also decreasing the spherical equivalent, sphere, and cylindrical components of the refractive error (Figure 13-2). Similar to synthetic segments, its effect depends on the thickness of the segment as well as the diameter and optic zone. The cornea follows the Barraquer and Blavatskaya postulates, which state that peripheral addition in the cornea causes flattening, and the diameter of the implanted ring determines the degree of flattening. Therefore, increasing the amount of tissue added, as well as decreasing the diameter, both cause a greater degree of myopia correction.[4] CAIRS implantation is also likely to have an additional beneficial biomechanical effect secondary to a redistribution of stress forces.

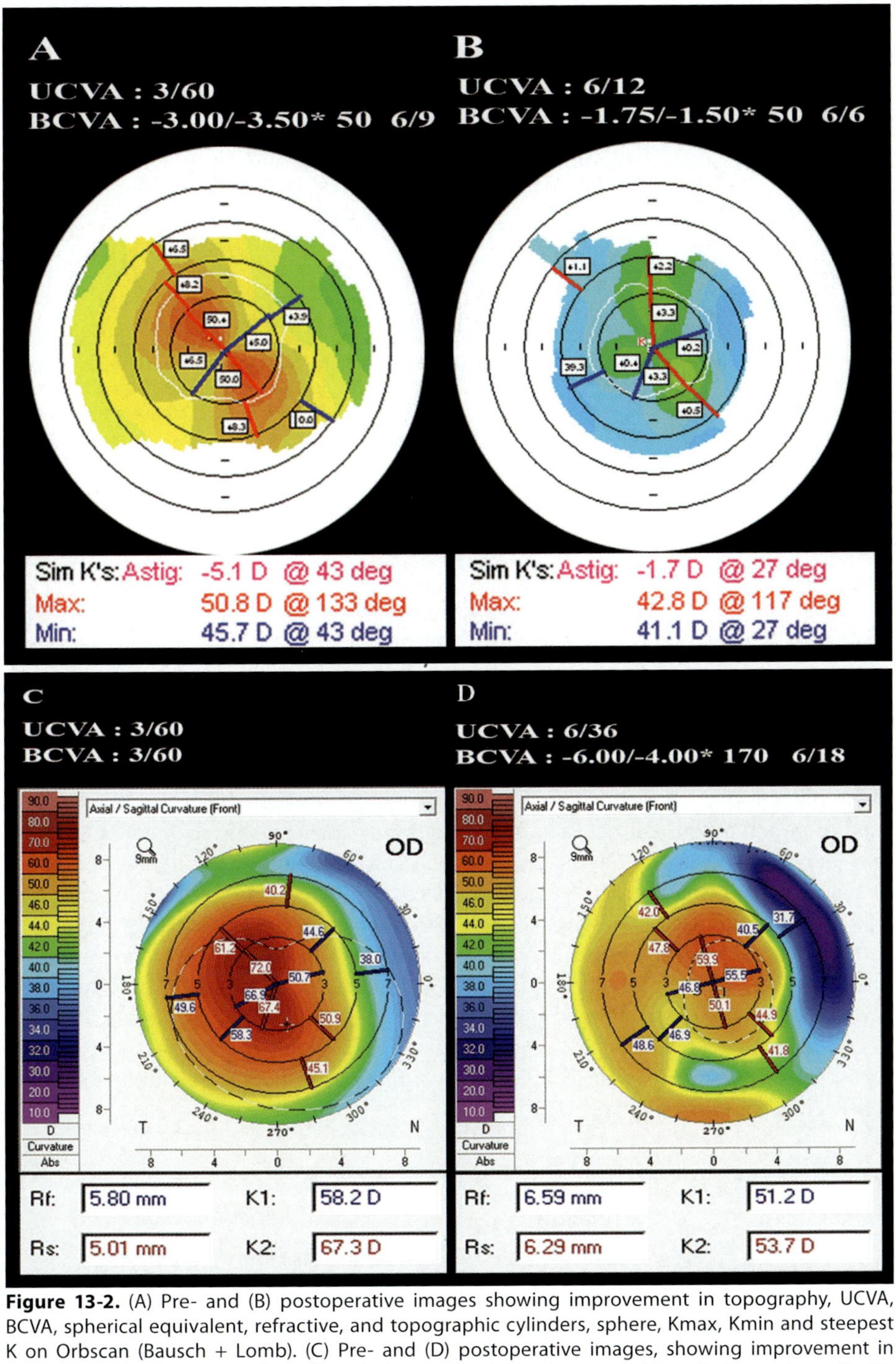

Figure 13-2. (A) Pre- and (B) postoperative images showing improvement in topography, UCVA, BCVA, spherical equivalent, refractive, and topographic cylinders, sphere, Kmax, Kmin and steepest K on Orbscan (Bausch + Lomb). (C) Pre- and (D) postoperative images, showing improvement in topography, UCVA, BCVA, spherical equivalent, refractive and topographic cylinders, sphere, K1, K2, on Pentacam (OCULUS).

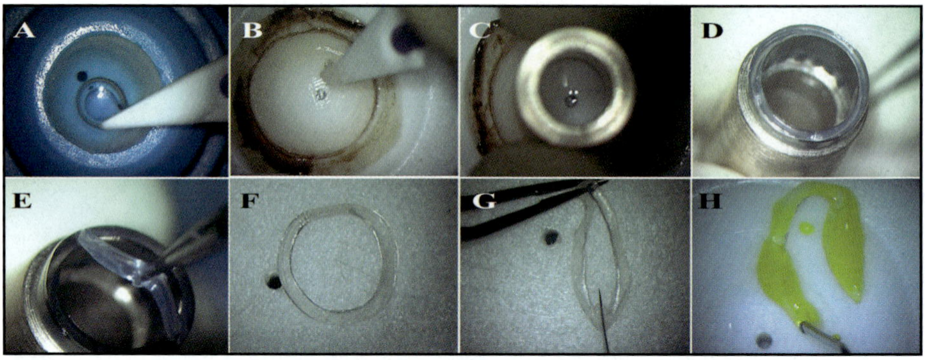

Figure 13-3. Preparation of CAIRS segments. (A, B) Epithelium and endothelium are completely removed from the donor corneal rim. (C-F) The Jacob CAIRS trephine is used to punch a ring segment of corneal stromal tissue of predetermined thickness. (G) The ring is cut to create either double segments or a single segment; (H) riboflavin is soaked on the tissue.

Technique

Screened and processed donor cornea is used to create corneal segments that are then implanted into the patient's cornea. Non-edematous donor corneal rims with negative serology for anti-HIV-1, anti-HIV-2, Hepatitis B surface antigen, anti–Hepatitis C virus, and venereal disease research laboratory test is utilized. The quality of the endothelium is not important as it is not transplanted. The donor cornea is first mounted on an artificial anterior chamber and epithelium removed completely. The center is then marked and laid upside down on a Teflon block, and the endothelium is removed as well. A double-bladed trephine designed by the author is then used to punch a segment of tissue from the donor cornea. This segment is then cut into 2 and soaked in riboflavin. Femtosecond laser–dissected channels are prepared in the patient's eye and the CAIRS segments are inserted into these channels either using the CAIRS inserter designed by the author or using curved 23-gauge forceps. In patients where progression is likely, this procedure is combined with corneal cross-linking (CXL) whereas in older patients, where only a regularization of topography is required, it can be performed in isolation. If indicated, CXL, either conventional or contact lens–assisted corneal cross-linking (CACXL; depending on the minimum corneal thickness) may be performed, either simultaneously or sequentially following CAIRS implantation (Figures 13-3 to 13-7).

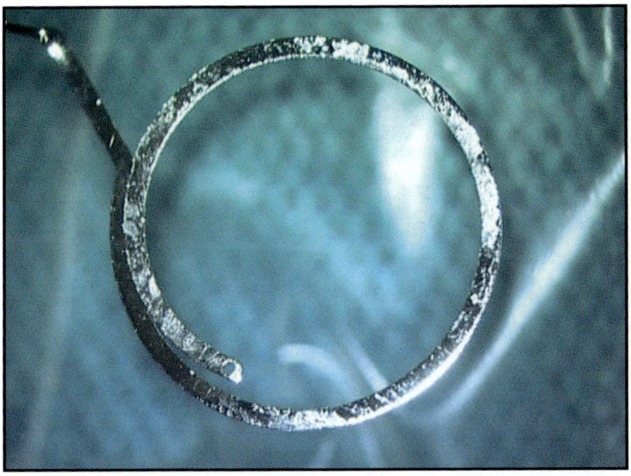

Figure 13-4. The Jacob CAIRS inserter is shown.

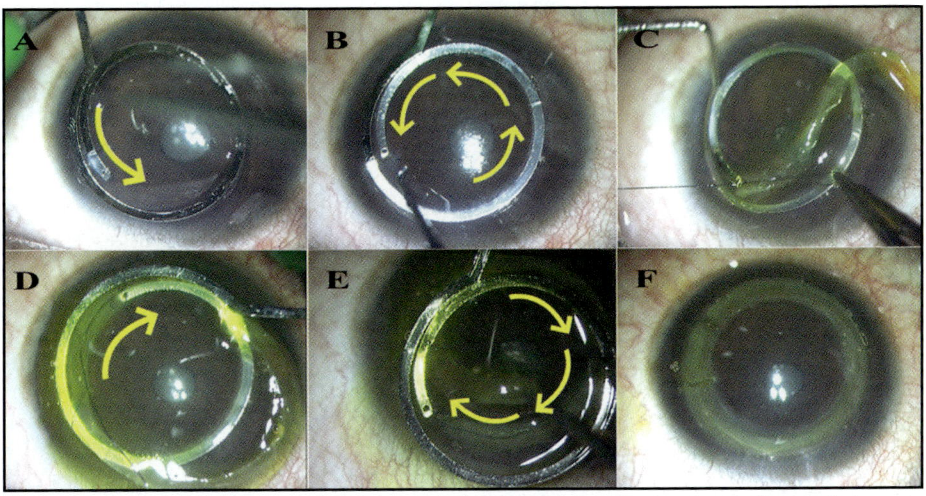

Figure 13-5. (A, B) The Jacob CAIRS inserter is introduced into femtosecond dissected channels created for CAIRS. (C) The segment is tied to the hole at the tip of the inserter using 8-0 nylon. (D, E) The inserter is withdrawn while simultaneously guiding the segment into the channel. (F) An almost 360° segment is seen lying within the channel.

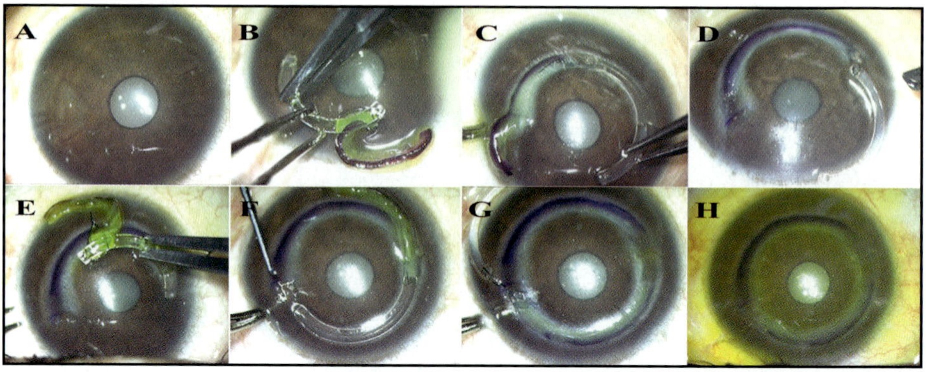

Figure 13-6. Implantation of CAIRS using an Intacs segment as a guide. (A) Femtosecond dissected channels are made in the patient's eye. (B) The CAIRS segment is tied to the positioning hole of the Intacs segment using 8-0 nylon. (C) Feeding the Intacs into the channel draws the CAIRS segment behind it. (D) The suture tying the CAIRS segment to the Intacs segment is cut and detached. (E-G) The same is repeated on the other side for implanting the second CAIRS segment. (H) Well-placed CAIRS segments are seen within the patient's stroma. CXL may be proceeded with if indicated.

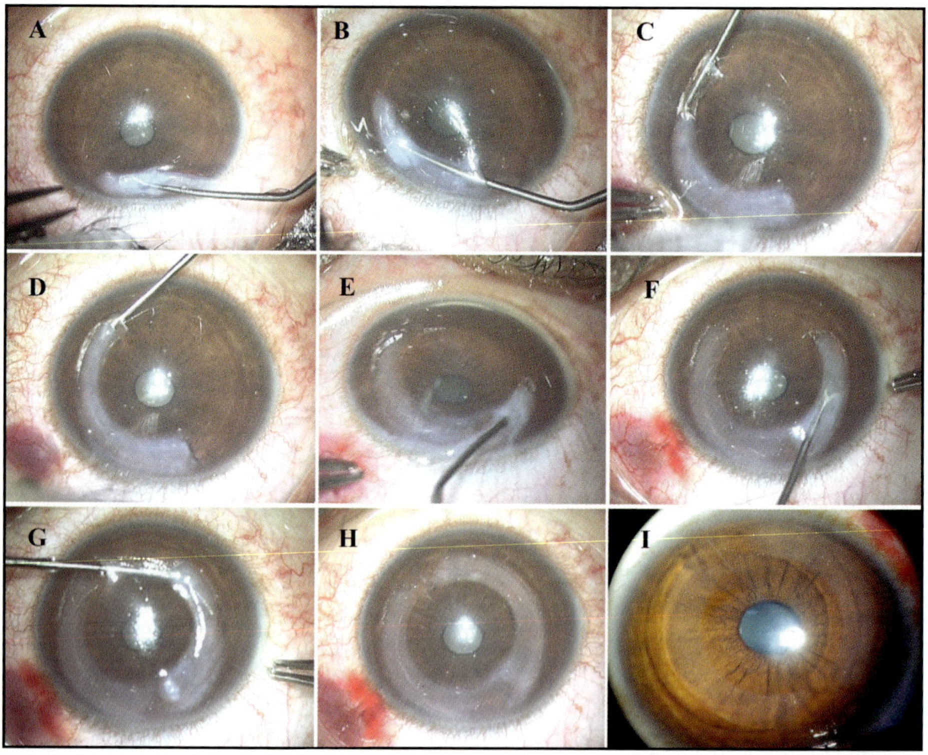

Figure 13-7. Implantation of CAIRS using a reverse Sinskey hook. (A, B) The CAIRS segment is introduced with a blunt rod into a femtosecond dissected channel. Care is taken to lay the segment out straight without any twists while inserting. (C, D) The CAIRS segment is engaged with a reverse Sinskey hook and pulled forward into position within the channel. (E-G) The same is repeated on the other side for implanting the second CAIRS segment; (H, I) well-placed CAIRS segments are seen within the patient's stroma. If indicated, proceed with CXL or CACXL.

Combining CAIRS With CACXL in Thin Corneas

Described by the author in 2013,[5,6] CACXL is used to safely perform CXL in patients with thin corneas (ie, for those who do not have at least 400 µm of minimum corneal thickness after epithelial removal). It works by increasing functional corneal thickness by placing a UV barrier-free soft contact lens soaked in riboflavin. This brings the UV irradiance at the plane of the endothelium to non-toxic levels in these thin corneas. A SofLens (Bausch + Lomb) daily disposable soft contact lens of negligible power and made of hilafilcon B with no UV filter is soaked in isotonic riboflavin solution for 30 minutes. This is performed simultaneous with the saturation of the deepithelialized cornea with riboflavin. Placing this riboflavin saturated soft contact lens over the corneal surface increases the functional corneal pachymetry by an additional thickness of approximately 100 µm contributed together by the soft contact lens (90 µm) and the precorneal riboflavin film. The minimum corneal pachymetry, after soaking in riboflavin, is measured again and the 100 µm of extra functional thickness that would be contributed to by the riboflavin soaked UV barrier free contact lens is added to this pachymetry. Once the combined pachymetry is confirmed to be 400 µm or above, either standard CXL at 3 mW/cm^2 for 30 minutes or accelerated CXL at 10 mW/cm^2 for 9 minutes (author's personal preference) is proceeded with. Accelerated protocol has added advantages of not only shortening the treatment time, but also decreasing intraoperative dehydration that may be caused by dextran-containing riboflavin.

CACXL, unlike hypoosmolar CXL is, therefore, not dependent on the swelling properties of the cornea, and functional corneal thickness is raised artificially by adding a riboflavin-saturated layer (thin precorneal riboflavin film, riboflavin-soaked barrier-free contact lens, and a thin pre–contact lens riboflavin film). Our published data showed a mean increase in thickness by 107.9 ± 9.4 µm (minimum 90 µm, which is the absolute thickness of the contact lens measured after riboflavin saturation) and this is generally sufficient for most thin corneas.[6] Sometimes, if very thin, corneas with 320 to 350 µm minimum corneal pachymetry do not attain a total functional pachymetry of 400 µm even after applying the soft contact lens. The principles of hypoosmolar and CACXL techniques may be combined. However, in this case, the advantage is that unlike conventional hypoosmolar CXL, a large amount of corneal swelling is not required as the contact lens already contributes to an increased thickness. A minimal increase in corneal thickness by applying a few drops of distilled water on the cornea is generally sufficient and is obtained easily and quickly. Therefore, this avoids the disadvantages of pure hypoosmolar technique, which requires large amount of swelling, causing ineffective CXL because of the widely separated collagen fibrils secondary to a larger degree of hydration and also has large inter- and intra-individual variation in corneal swelling properties with failure to attain desired swelling in some patients resulting in having to abort.

CACXL decreases UV transmittance to approximately 60% to 70% at the stromal level. This was sufficient in our study, with no patient showing signs of progression.

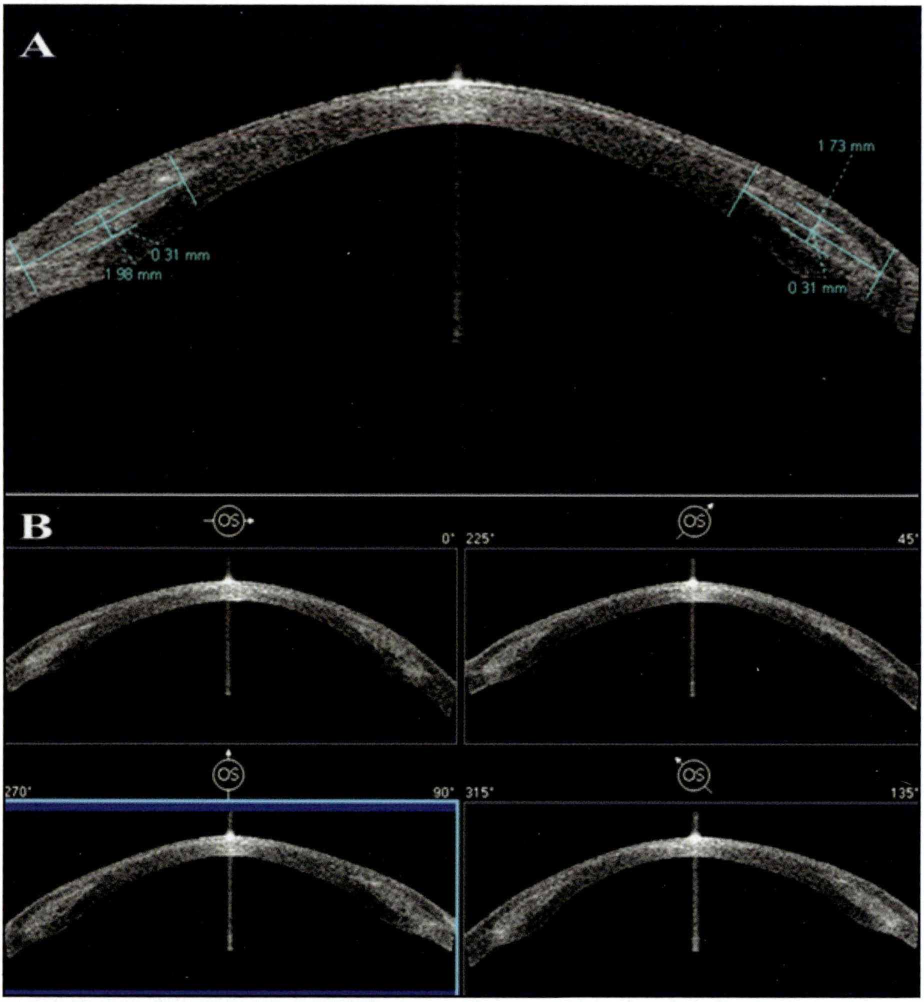

Figure 13-8. (A, B) Well-positioned CAIRS segments are seen on anterior segment optical coherence tomography. Depth of placement is about 50% of minimum corneal thickness. Surrounding host tissue is quiet with lack of reaction, inflammation, or edema.

Clinical effects in the form of sufficiently deep demarcation line is seen (Figure 13-8). In addition, it has been shown that the biomechanical efficacy of collagen CXL is higher in thin corneas as compared to thick corneas due to increased oxygen availability.[7]

It is important not to select a contact lens with built-in UV barrier for this technique. This may be tested for by using a digital UV meter as well as by checking product literature. Contact lenses made of narafilcon A and senofilcon A have the highest blockage and the lowest transmittance, whereas hilafilcon B, filcon IV, nelfilcon A, enfilcon A, lotrafilcon A, and lotrafilcon B have the highest UVA transmittance.[8]

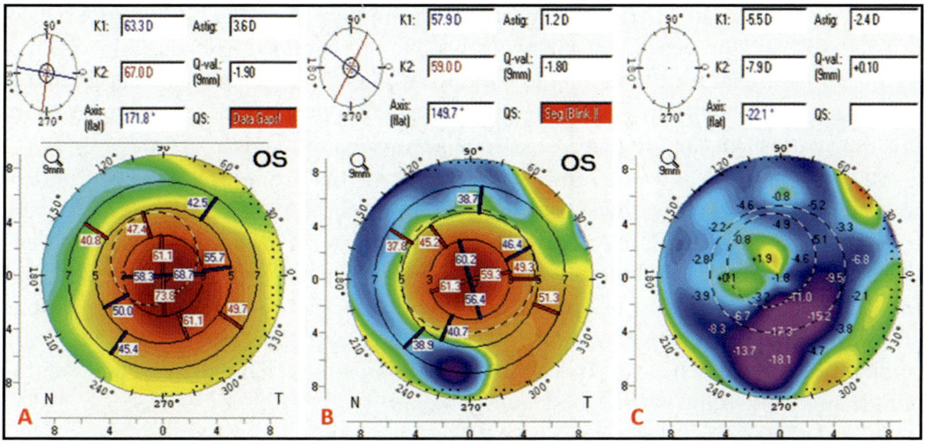

Figure 13-9. CAIRS with CACXL performed for a patient with Kmax of 76.7 D and thinnest pachymetry of 390 µm, for whom normally a DALK would have been indicated. Good results are seen in uncorrected-distance visual acuity (UDVA) and corrected-distance visual acuity. A well-placed segment is seen on anterior segment optical coherence tomography and flattening and regularization of the cone are seen on comparing the pre-and postoperative topographical maps.

Though these other UV transmitting contact lenses may be used, the author does not have personal experience with them.

Use in Corneas That Are Steep but Not Thin Enough to Warrant DALK

Deep anterior lamellar keratoplasty (DALK) is usually indicated in patients who have corneas that are too thin and/or steep to crosslink safely. An increased risk of complications has been reported in corneas steeper than 58 diopters (D) following CXL and, therefore, such corneas undergo DALK despite sometimes having sufficient thickness to safely crosslink. In the published study series, the initial flattening produced by the CAIRS allowed us to safely crosslink patients up to 67.4 D without an increased incidence of haze, scarring, or other complications.[2] Subsequently we have done steeper corneas as well. Figure 13-9 shows CAIRS with CXL done in a cornea with preoperative Kmax of 76.7 D.

Advantages and Other Considerations

This is a simple procedure that has shown safety, efficacy, and stability over time and can be used for treatment of keratoconus and other corneal ectatic conditions. It gives significant improvement in UDVA, spectacle corrected-distance visual acuity, spherical equivalent, and topographic parameters. Unlike synthetic ICRS, which require a minimum pachymetry of 450 µm in the zone of implantation to prevent erosion and extrusion, CAIRS do not need to be implanted at 80% depth and we have utilized 50% to 70% depth placement for producing an effect. Eye rubbing, which is a common complaint in keratoconic patients, is also likely to have a lesser effect on allogenic than on synthetic segments. We had no complications of extrusion, erosion, melt, or necrosis of the segments or corneal stroma in our series.

Stromal rejection is a potential disadvantage of this procedure; however, understandably, the risk is even lower than in DALK, which by itself has a low risk as well, because of the lower volume of stromal transfer, absence of epithelial or endothelial transfer, early repopulation of the tissue from all sides by host keratocytes, and implantation only in mid-peripheral zone with complete sparing over the pupillary axis. Further deantigenization is possible by using processed tissue. Allogenic implants also already have been described for use in aphakia, hypermetropia, keratoconus, and presbyopia with a good safety track.[9,10]

References

1. Kanellopoulos AJ, Pe LH, Perry HD, et al. Modified intracorneal ring segment implantations (INTACS) for the management of moderate to advanced keratoconus: efficacy and complications. *Cornea*. 2006;25:29-33
2. Jacob S, Patel SR, Agarwal A, Ramalingam A, Saijimol AI, Raj JM. Corneal allogenic intrastromal ring segments (CAIRS) combined with corneal cross-linking for keratoconus. *J Refract Surg*. 2018;34(5):296-303.
3. Jacob S. CAIRS A new technique for keratoconus and corneal ecstasias [video]. YouTube. https://www.youtube.com/watch?v=qF-9ycSQPq8. Published May 9, 2017. Accessed October 2, 2018.
4. Barraquer JI. Modification of refraction by means of intracorneal inclusion. *Int Ophthamol Clin*. 1966;6(1):53-78.
5. Mazzotta C, Jacob S, Agarwal A, Kumar DA. In vivo confocal microscopy after contact lens-assisted corneal collagen cross-linking for thin keratoconic corneas. *J Refract Surg*. 2016;32(5):326-331.
6. Jacob S, Kumar DA, Agarwal A, Basu S, Sinha P, Agarwal A. Contact lens-assisted collagen cross-linking (CACXL): a new technique for cross-linking thin corneas. *J Refract Surg*. 2014;30(6):366-372.
7. Kling S, Richoz O, Hammer A, Tabibian D, Jacob S, Agarwal A, Hafezi F. Increased biomechanical efficacy of corneal cross-linking in thin corneas due to higher oxygen availability. *J Refract Surg*. 2015;31(12):840-846.
8. Bilgihan K, Yuksel E, Deniz NG, Yuksel N. Can possible toxic effect of ultraviolet-A after corneal cross-linking be prevented? In vitro transmittance study of contact lenses at 370 nm wavelength. *Cutan Ocul Toxicol*. 2014;34(4):271-275.
9. Jacob S, Kumar DA, Agarwal A, Basu S, Sinha P, Agarwal A. Contact lens-assisted collagen cross-linking (CACXL): a new technique for cross-linking thin corneas. *J Refract Surg*. 2014;30(6):366-372.
10. Pradhan KR, Reinstein DZ, Carp GI, Archer TJ, Gobbe M, Gurung R. Femtosecond laser-assisted keyhole endokeratophakia: correction of hyperopia by implantation of an allogeneic lenticule obtained by SMILE from a myopic donor. *J Refract Surg*. 2013;29(11):777-82.

Please see videos on the accompanying website at
www.healio.com/books/DALKvideos

Video Appendix
Pre-Descemetic DALK Video

Lim Li, MBBS, FRCS(Ed), MMed(Ophth), FAMS(S'pore)

Mastering DALK: A Video Textbook on Deep Anterior Lamellar Keratoplasty offers this video appendix online only.

Please see videos on the accompanying website at
www.healio.com/books/DALKvideos

Jacob S, ed. *Mastering DALK: A Video Textbook on Deep Anterior Lamellar Keratoplasty* (pp 167).

Financial Disclosures

Dr. Sriram Annavajjhala has no financial or proprietary interest in the materials presented herein.

Dr. Harkaran Bains has no financial or proprietary interest in the materials presented herein.

Dr. Rénuka S. Birbal has no financial or proprietary interest in the materials presented herein.

Dr. Alan N. Carlson has no financial or proprietary interest in the materials presented herein.

Dr. Melissa B. Daluvoy has no financial or proprietary interest in the materials presented herein.

Dr. Vittoria De Rosa has no financial or proprietary interest in the materials presented herein.

Dr. Alaa M. Eldanasoury is a consultant for STAAR Surgical, NIDEK Co, and PhysIOL.

Dr. Ronald N. Gaster has no financial or proprietary interest in the materials presented herein.

Dr. Noopur Gupta has no financial or proprietary interest in the materials presented herein.

Dr. Kristin E. Hirabayashi has no financial or proprietary interest in the materials presented herein.

Dr. Soosan Jacob has a patent pending for shaped corneal segments and devices and processes used to manufacture them.

Dr. Bennie H. Jeng has no financial or proprietary interest in the materials presented herein.

Dr. Bina John has no financial or proprietary interest in the materials presented herein.

Dr. Terry Kim has no financial or proprietary interest in the materials presented herein.

Dr. Lim Li has no financial or proprietary interest in the materials presented herein.

Dr. Charles C. Lin has no financial or proprietary interest in the materials presented herein.

Dr. Prafulla Maharana has no financial or proprietary interest in the materials presented herein.

Dr. Gerrit R. J. Melles is a consultant for DORC International/Dutch Ophthalmic USA and SurgiCube International.

Dr. Sujatha Mohan has no financial or proprietary interest in the materials presented herein.

Dr. Smita Narasimhan has no financial or proprietary interest in the materials presented herein.

Dr. Ashiyana Nariani has no financial or proprietary interest in the materials presented herein.

Dr. Jack Parker is a consultant for DORC International/Dutch Ophthalmic USA and Ziemer Ophthalmic Systems.

Dr. Mukesh Patil has no financial or proprietary interest in the materials presented herein.

Dr. Claudia Perez-Straziota has no financial or proprietary interest in the materials presented herein.

Dr. Pranita Sahay has no financial or proprietary interest in the materials presented herein.

Areeckal Incy Saijimol has no financial or proprietary interest in the materials presented herein.

Dr. Namrata Sharma has no financial or proprietary interest in the materials presented herein.

Dr. Deepali Singhal has no financial or proprietary interest in the materials presented herein.

Dr. T. Suchi Smitha has no financial or proprietary interest in the materials presented herein.

Prof. Leopoldo Spadea has no financial or proprietary interest in the materials presented herein.

Dr. Rishi Swarup has no financial or proprietary interest in the materials presented herein.

Dr. Radhika Tandon has no financial or proprietary interest in the materials presented herein.

Dr. Sherif Said Tolees has no financial or proprietary interest in the materials presented herein.

Dr. C. Maya Tong has no financial or proprietary interest in the materials presented herein.

Dr. Korine van Dijk has no financial or proprietary interest in the materials presented herein.

Dr. Murugesan Vanathi has no financial or proprietary interest in the materials presented herein.

Index